THE MANAGEMENT OF HOME CARE SERVICES

Stephen Crystal was principal investigator of the Home Care Fiscal Management Project and director of the Center for Human Services Research and Development in New York City's Human Resources Administration. Dr. Crystal is now Associate Research Professor and Director, Division on Aging at Rutgers University's Institute for Health, Health Care Policy, and Aging Research.

Camilla Flemming was Project Director of the Home Care Fiscal Management Project. She is now Project Manager in the New York City Human Resources Administration's Office of Program Development and principal investigator of Project GAIN: Greater Access to Independence for Homeless and Foster Care Youth.

Pearl Beck was Research Director for the Project and is Project Manager in the New York City Human Resources Administration's Office of Policy and Economic Research.

Geraldine Smolka participated in the Project as consultant on the staff of the Nova Institute in New York City. She is now at Blue Cross/Blue Shield of Massachusetts.

THE MANAGEMENT OF HOME CARE SERVICES

**Stephen Crystal
Camilla Flemming
Pearl Beck
Geraldine Smolka**

**and the Home Care Fiscal Management
Consortium**

SPRINGER PUBLISHING COMPANY
New York

Springer Publishing Company, Inc.
536 Broadway
New York, NY 10012

87 88 89 90 91 / 5 4 3 2 1

Library of Congress Cataloging-in-Publication Data

The Management of home care services.

"This book is a revision and extension of the final report of the Home Care Fiscal Management Project"—Pref.
Bibliography: p.
Includes index.
1. Home care services—Administration.   2. Home care services—United States—Administration—Case studies.
3. Home Care Fiscal Management Project (New York, N.Y.)
I. Crystal, Stephen, 1946-   .   II. Home Care Fiscal Management Project (New York, N.Y.)   [DNLM: 1. Home Care Services—economics—United States.   2. Home Care Services—organization & administration—United States.
WY 115 M2665]
RA645.3.M36   1987   362.1′4′068   87–12929
ISBN 0-8261-5660-6

Printed in the United States of America

Contents

Preface

This book is a revision and extension of the final report of the Home Care Fiscal Management Project. The Project grew out of a concern that the rapid growth and expansion of home care programs has not always been paralleled by the implementation of effective techniques to manage and control service operations and funds. Program growth has often outstripped the ability of states and localities to achieve efficiency and accountability in delivering services. While effective management control practices have been developed in some places, there has been little sharing of knowledge about these improvements among state and local governments. Thus, states and localities administering home care programs often have found themselves reinventing the same wheels in developing solutions to very similar programmatic and financial management problems.

New York City, operator of the largest single home care program in the country, was particularly concerned with these problems, and through its Center for Human Services Research and Development (CHSRD) received a grant from the U.S. Department of Health and Human Services. The grant, which funded the Home Care Fiscal Management Project, was supported by the Administration on Aging, the Administration for Developmental Disabilities, and the Office of Policy Development of the Office of Human Development Services. The project was headed by Stephen Crystal, Director of the CHSRD (within the city's Human Resources Administration) and Principal Investigator of the project. Day-to-day administration of the project was the responsibility of Camilla Flemming, Project Director. Ms. Flemming was supported by Pearl Beck, who oversaw the publication of the final report, edited and published the project newsletter, served as Research Director of the project, and later served as Project Director.

The project sought to identify innovative public fiscal management practices in home care and to provide access to information on these practices to those who provide or contract for home care services. Dissemination of information on effective fiscal management practices was aimed at providing the basis for better-informed program management and more judicious use of home care dollars. The project's objectives were (1) to identify effective home care fiscal and program management practices in use in local and state jurisdictions across the country, (2) to form a consortium of five states and localities that had developed especially effective or innovative practices and that were willing to provide technical assistance to other state and local governments, and (3) to disseminate information on these and other home care practices through workshops, videotapes, newsletters, and publications.

Governments were invited and agreed to join New York City in a consortium. Consortium participants (in addition to New York City) were Alameda County in California and the states of Connecticut, Texas, and Washington. These four were chosen after a review of current home care fiscal management practices in state and local governments across the nation. They were selected primarily because they offered practices for dissemination that were innovative and apparently effective and represented diverse administrative, delivery, and provider structures. The group included participants from the major geographic regions of the nation. Consortium members collaborated with project staff in project training sessions, the project newsletter, and the development of documentation on their agencies' practices.

To encourage the direct or modified adoption of improved management techniques among states and localities, the project conducted workshops throughout the country in 1984. These workshops provided information on other states' fiscal management practices. In addition, individual consortium members presented their techniques at professional conferences. Project support in some cases also assisted consortium participants in further development of their practices, such as the development of a budget planning module in the Alameda County system.

In each jurisdiction one official functioned as the lead consortium representative, participating actively in training sessions that explained his or her agency's practices and drafting the descriptions of agency practices that are the heart of Part II of this book. Staff of New York City's Nova Institute acted as consultants to the project. Nova's President, David A. Grossman, provided overall supervision for Nova's work on this project. Nova's principal involvement in the project was in the persons of Geraldine Smolka and Bruce A. Gombos. Eugene Shinn of the National HomeCaring Council also was a consultant to the project, focusing on cost analysis. These individuals are listed in the roster of consortium members.

While material that became chapters of this book was drafted by different project participants, the volume as a whole represents a truly collaborative effort. The innovative management practices described were identified through a national solicitation conducted by the project staff. Management issues in home care were discussed in initial meetings of consortium members and project staff, producing a cooperative approach to defining the issues in home care management, informed by in-depth expertise of a variety of quite different local management approaches. Project staff revised and edited the material drafted by consortium participants.

Descriptions and analyses that became chapters of the book were developed by Stephen Crystal, Camilla Flemming, Bruce Gombos, Eugene Shinn, Tom McCormick, Louis Goldblatt, Ernest McKenney, Kathy Leitch, Kathryn Haslanger, and Geraldine Smolka. Eve McCormick, an HRA summer intern, carried out research on practices in nonconsortium states, which is drawn on in Chapter 11. The original final report was substantially restructured and revised for book publication with the development of the new Preface and Chapter 1 by Stephen Crystal and Camilla Flemming; with the addition of new chapters (4 and 5) on personnel and independent contractors prepared by Camilla Flemming; and with additions to other chapters by Stephen Crystal.

OVERVIEW OF THE BOOK

The issues discussed in this study may seem at first glance to be relatively technical administrative problems. Yet they are crucial for the cost-effective delivery and indeed for the viability and growth of home care, and so are vital for the care of the elderly and disabled.

Part I provides, in Chapter 1, an overview of the home care system. In the second chapter, on fiscal management, the effort is to place the issues for home care in the context of a broader analysis of state and local fiscal structures and procedures, focusing particularly on the effort to integrate fiscal and programmatic information and control systems. Integration is presented as a key objective for management improvement, particularly for such functions as budgeting, accounting, performance measurement, audit, programmatic statistics, and monitoring of client characteristics and needs.

Understanding the cost structure of home care services is of obvious importance to home care administrators. To date, there has been a surprisingly wide degree of variation in defining what costs have been included, how the costs should be calculated, and what standard quantity of service should be used to compare costs. Chapter 3 reviews the problem of cost analysis in home care, providing examples of how unit costing is carried out in several jurisdictions.

Part I also includes chapters on personnel practices in home care and on employer–employee relationships in independent provider programs, two crucial current issues in home care management. These issues are especially important because quality of service in home care depends predominantly on the performance and attitude of individual workers who provide services in a setting remote from day-to-day supervision, often at rates little above the minimum wage. Home care is among the most labor-intensive of the human services; payments to direct-service workers for salary and benefits typically account for 80 to 95 percent of total program costs. Problems of provider recruitment, training, supervision, compensation, and turnover are thus crucial to home care. Chapter 4 discusses these problems.

The nature of the employer–employee relationship in programs that use independent providers or family members is explored in Chapter 5. Many home care programs utilize vendor agencies under contract with governmental funding agencies to employ, pay, and supervise the actual workers, while relatively few use public employees as providers. In a considerable number of programs, the worker is considered an independent provider. Though some large programs such as New York City's have moved away from this practice, independent provider arrangements still represent a central issue in home care administration. Such arrangements can minimize program administrative costs and help to make home care cost-effective and therefore financially and politically feasible even where substantial numbers of hours per week are required. They can also maximize the degree of autonomy and control accruing to the client receiving service, a factor particularly valued by some client subgroups such as the nonelderly disabled. On the other hand, such arrangements can create the potential for worker exploitation and can create serious ambiguities of legal status, responsibility, and accountability in the relationships among worker, client, and funding agency. Is a *de facto* or common-law employment relationship created in such situations, either between the worker and client or worker and funding agency? Who, if anyone, is responsible for payments of Social Security, unemployment insurance, disability payments, and other benefits, or for income tax withholding? What is the status of family members paid to care for their relatives (not an uncommon practice in home care programs)? These are among the questions taken up in Chapter 5.

Part II applies the themes discussed in Part I to specific local and state programs, describing the management practices of the five consortium members (Chapters 6 through 10). These program descriptions provide several important models for integrating fiscal and programmatic information and control systems; achieving more rational and equitable program and service allocation decisions through use of information systems; and effectively managing the contractual and financial relationships between government agencies responsible for funding and supervising programs and the nonprofit or proprietary provider agencies commonly responsible for the actual delivery of services under governmental contract. The book ends with Chapter 11, which reviews these practices and the approaches of other states and localities in light of the themes described in the preceding chapters.

As home care takes on an increasingly central role in the long-term care system, it becomes more and more important that these programs be managed efficiently. The aging of the population and a shift away from reliance on institutional care are increasing the need and demand for home care services, but justifying allocation of additional resources demands that programs demonstrate managerial credibility. Developments in information technology create new opportunities for more sophisticated approaches to integrated information management and program control, but too often administrators lack information about the state of the art as a starting point for improving their own management systems. We hope that the information in this book will help to provide solutions to the complex problems faced by those responsible for providing these services.

Acknowledgments

Special thanks are due to the following persons from across the country who provided additional information: Helen Drake, Phoenix Aging Services Division; Lucian Shockey, Arkansas Department of Human Services; Greg McKinney, Georgia Department of Medical Assistance; Sheri Mize-Wrightman, Illinois Department of Aging; Nola Aalberts, Iowa Department of Health; Sabra Burdick, Maine Department of Human Services; Ellen Leiserson, Maryland Department of Human Resources; Robert Mollica, Massachusetts Executive Office on Aging; James Nye, Michigan Department of Social Services; Elaine Reiter, Missouri Division of Aging; Rowena Bopp, New Jersey Department of Human Services; Ted Taberski, New York City Department for the Aging; Anita Waters, Office of Home Care Services, New York City Human Resources Administration; Ann Hallock, New York State Department of Social Services; Mary Jo Littlewood, Wake County (North Carolina) Council on Aging; Doris Stohl, Oklahoma Department of Human Services; David Herr and Dan McGuire, Pennsylvania Department of Aging; Ray Rickard, South Dakota Department of Social Services; Sharon Boatman, Texas Department of Human Resources; Ted Mable, Vermont

Human Services Agency; Emily Layzer, New York, New York; Rick Zawadski, On Lok Senior Health Services; Janet Nasif, New York, New York; Jeanne Farrell and Pamela Booth, National HomeCaring Council; Brian Burwell, Systemetrics, Inc.; Eileen O'Neill, Boston, Massachusetts; Michael Power, Arthur Young and Company; Pamela Doty, Health Care Financing Administration; Robert Ficke, National Association of State Units on Aging; and Toshio Totora, American Public Welfare Association.

The Home Care Fiscal Management Project and this book also benefited from the support of the principal administrators of the New York City Human Resources Administration. We thank especially Robert Trobe, who was HRA Deputy Administrator, for his support in the often challenging endeavor of operating a research center carrying out national-level and consortium projects within a municipal agency. We also thank former HRA Administrator Jack Krauskopf for his aid, and Carol Raphael, Director of the New York City Office of Home Care Services and subsequently Deputy Administrator for Medical Assistance, for her cooperation and contributions to the training and publications.

The Home Care Fiscal Management Consortium

Louis Goldblatt represented Connecticut in the Consortium as Manager of Program Development in that state's Department on Aging.

Bruce Gombos, who was a consultant at the Nova Institute, is Director of Financial Planning for the New York City Health and Hospitals Corporation.

Kathryn Haslanger is Assistant Deputy Administrator for Program Budget Control in the Medical Assistance Program of New York City's Human Resources Administration.

Kathy Leitch was Supervisor of Area Agency on Aging Operations in the State of Washington's Department of Social and Health Services, and subsequently Special Assistant to the Director of that agency's Bureau of Aging and Adult Services.

Tom McCormick represented Alameda County, California, in the Consortium. He is Director of Adult Services for the Alameda County Social Services Agency.

Ernest McKenney represented Texas in the Consortium as Director of In-Home Services, Provider Services Branch, Services to Aged and Disabled in the Texas Department of Human Services.

Eugene Shinn, previously with the National HomeCaring Council, is Director of the Research and Demonstration Center at the Graduate School of Social Service at Fordham University, New York City.

THE MANAGEMENT OF
HOME CARE SERVICES

PART I
Toward Improved
Management and Control

1

The Home Care System

What is home care, and who does it serve? What lies behind its rapid expansion? How is it funded and administered? To set the stage for the succeeding discussion, this chapter outlines answers to these questions and introduces some of the basic programmatic and fiscal management issues.

IN-HOME SERVICES AND LONG-TERM CARE

Home care is among the most complex and administratively challenging services delivered by states and localities; it is also among the most important for the welfare of aged, disabled, and other physically impaired persons. The success of human service providers and government in managing home care in a cost-effective and efficient manner will do much to determine whether the greatly needed transition—from the present, institutionally biased, long-term care system to a balanced system using institutionalization as a last rather than a first resort—can progress.

Long-term care of impaired persons, especially the elderly, accounts for a large and increasing share of total expenditures for health care and related services. For example, institutional and home-based long-term care accounted for an estimated 48%

of Medicaid spending in 1983 (Doty, Liu, & Wiener, 1985), a proportion that appears to have remained relatively stable since 1979. To some, the term *long-term care* mostly brings to mind nursing homes, yet in-home services now represent a substantial and increasing share. The historical predominance of the nursing home in long-term care represents in part financing biases built into the major health care financing programs, which in turn reflect in part a very realistic legislative and administrative concern with the potential costs of in-home benefits.

The predominance of nursing homes in publicly financed long-term care—with expenditures estimated at as much as 10 times those for in-home care—has never reflected the distribution of care needs. A substantial body of experience and research now indicates that care can be provided safely and satisfactorily at home for persons with a wide range of impairment levels and care needs, including those typical of many people currently in nursing homes (Reif & Trager, 1985; Hughes, 1986). Such care is considerably more satisfying for the great majority of its recipients, and it is less expensive than institutional care on a per-person basis, in most cases. This does not necessarily mean, however, that its expansion can be accompanied by reductions in total long-term care expenditures (Weissert, 1985a). Many elderly have difficulty in adapting late in life to removal from a home they may have lived in for many decades and to institutionalization. There can be devastating effects on morale or even on survival. As more attention has come to be paid to these problems, greater emphasis has been placed on the development of in-home care.

In most European countries, in-home care has long been financed by government on comparable terms to the financing of institutional care (Reif & Trager, 1985). Home care was slower to develop in the United States. In recent years, however, these services have experienced major development, often outstripping the administrative systems that grew like Topsy to support them. Thus, for example, New York City's Home Attendant Program evolved as a small-scale system of two-party special-grant welfare checks provided to clients receiving or eligible for Aid to the Aged, Blind or Disabled, prior to that program's federalization in 1974. By the mid-1980s it had grown to a half-billion-dollar operation. The evolution from administrative systems oriented toward cash welfare payments to the complex and specialized service delivery system described in Chapter 10 required major reorganization and administrative restructuring over an extended period.

Recent years have witnessed a dramatic upsurge in the scope of home care, with annual growth estimated at 20 to 25% (Waldo, Levit, & Lazenby, 1986). Between 1974 and 1983 home health payments under Medicaid increased from $31 million to $597 million, an 1800% increase. In the same years, Medicare payments for such services rose from $119 million to $1.5 billion (Doty, Liu, & Wiener, 1985). By 1985, Medicare payments had increased further to $2.2 billion, reflecting strong underlying demand for in-home care, even under the severely restricted and time-limited terms of the Medicare benefit (Leader, 1986). Approximately 5 percent of Medicare beneficiaries used the benefit in 1983, double the 1974 proportion, but they averaged only 26 visits per user (Bishop & Stassen, 1986; Cornick, 1985). For the longer term, supportive home care programs that are the principal subject of this book, demand has been great and increasing, though often unsatisfied. The majority of the estimated $6.3 billion cost to all payers in 1985 was paid out of pocket by patients and their families (Waldo, Levit, & Lazenby, 1986), creating severe financial burdens on them and new pressures for expansion of publicly financed programs. Title XX of the Social Security Act and Title III of the Older Americans Act are principal funding sources, along with Medicaid in a few states and increasing amounts of unreimbursed state funds. Demand for these services is such that some states, such as California, supplement Title XX home care funds with as much as hundreds of millions of dollars in state funds. Since 1982, in some states, nontechnical home care under Medicaid has been expanded through home and community-based waivers. In addition to the rapid growth under these programs, home care funded by other federal and state programs has also been increasing. Altogether, public and private costs are projected to increase to $11 billion by 1990 (Frost & Sullivan, 1983).

Local and state agencies have found ways to generate federal reimbursement for substantial parts, if not all, of their home care expenditures, through often creative uses of federal matching programs and through block grants, but there has been little federal leadership in developing a national system of home care. Indeed, there has been a great deal of federal reticence and resistance to permitting basic health financing programs to meet any significant portions of the extensive need and demand for home

care. Indeed, while manifest needs have pressed states to develop often extensive systems, federal entitlements, such as Medicare's home health benefit, have in some cases become more
restrictive, while proposed federal initiatives on catastrophic
care have excluded in-home and other long-term care. State and
local initiatives have been heterogeneous in almost every key
respect, from program auspices to structure to scope of services
provided. For some clients in some jurisdictions, this state of
affairs means lack of access to needed care and excessive reliance on institutional solutions to long-term care problems, as
well as inefficiency and duplicative effort. On the more positive
side, it has fostered administrative innovation and created a series of "natural experiments" with alternative ways of organiz-
ing services. To learn from these opportunities, however, dissemination and analysis of these alternative administrative
approaches is essential.

While the scope of home care programs is already large, the
potential for organized, large-scale benefit systems is even
greater but depends crucially on development of efficient, equitable means for administering them in a cost-effective manner.
Private insurance, for example, thus far plays a very limited role
in financing long-term home care, but insurers and insurance
regulators face increasing pressures to make such benefits available. Existing models for home care delivery have not inspired
confidence on the part of insurers. Expansion of the Medicare
benefit to provide for long-term, supportive home care for the
chronically impaired has been widely advocated. Any such initiatives would require development of administrative and financial systems that provide a basis for efficient program management, cost control, and management of relationships among
multiple organizations involved in the financing and actual delivery of care—in short, the kinds of problems discussed in this
book. Thus, improving the state of the art in managing home
care systems is important not only in the efficient management
of existing systems but as a basis for further development of the
home care alternative. The continued aging of the population—
in particular the growth of the 75-and-older age cohort, which
has a much higher rate of demand for long-term and in-home
care—further expands the potential market and need.

The efforts at improving the management of home care described in this book vary widely, but they share the objective of
making more rational the organization and delivery of a set of

services that tend to be fragmented because they operate in a complex and fragmented legislative, regulatory, and financial setting. Home care services are in many respects the stepchild of health care in the United States. Yet, despite the emphasis in national health legislation on acute care, long-term care services have been too important and too badly needed to be ignored. Legislative provisions originally intended as limited and ancillary benefits have been expanded in the face of high demand for services. States have made creative use of nonspecific enabling authorities in federal legislation, as with the "social services" provisions of the Social Security Act, first under Titles IV and XVI and later under Title XX, and with the use by New York and some other states of ambiguous "personal care" provisions in the Medicaid statute, Title XIX. Home care has often grown through local and state initiative and the application of a wide variety of funding sources, as reflected in many of the service models described in this book. The result has been a system whose complexity and diversity almost defy description. There has been a chronic lack of any central compilation of data on programs administered in hundreds of different ways, and under hundreds of different auspices. Information is scarce about such basic matters as the current cost of home care services nationally, and the number and characteristics of persons served.

A series of converging developments have increased demand for home care services. These include, especially, fundamental changes in hospital reimbursement systems designed to reduce sharply the length of stay and to limit stays to the amount of time necessary to provide specialized, acute care. Meanwhile, the availability of nursing home beds has declined as bed supplies fail to keep pace with the demand generated by (1) the increased numbers of elderly persons; (2) the "aging" of the elderly population, within which the oldest age groups have been growing much more quickly than the "young-old" (65 to 74 years) population; and (3) the decreased availability of family care as more adult women enter the workplace. Nursing home admission screening procedures have been widely implemented, squeezing out many elderly who do not need skilled nursing care or constant attendance but who nevertheless cannot remain safely at home without help. In fact, many of the screening systems appear to assume implicitly that some form of home care is available, justifying this rejection for nursing home care patients whose need is "merely" for assistance with basic activities of daily living.

As patients are discharged "quicker and sicker" from hospitals and have increasing difficulty in gaining access to nursing homes, either for convalescent care or longer-term help, new challenges are set before the home care system. On the one hand, the increasing presence of very sick individuals with specialized care needs places an increasing demand on provider agencies to provide access to "high-tech" home care services. Patients with specialized care needs—including total parenteral nutrition, injected medications, catheter care, monitoring of complex regimes of powerful medications, and intravenous lines—are increasingly referred to home care. At the same time, programs must cope with a patient load that increasingly needs extensive care with basic activities of daily living, with the need for the availability of a helper for many hours a day or even continuously. While the high-tech care needs appear to call for specialized, highly skilled care involving a highly trained and therefore costly care provider, the extensive personal care that is also often needed would be prohibitively expensive to provide except through relatively "low-tech," nonspecialized care providers of the sort traditionally characteristic of the state and locally administered programs. The obvious implication of all of this is that there is an increasing need to integrate better a range of services and caregivers, in order to assure that appropriately coordinated care is provided to vulnerable patients. The mechanisms for this coordination of care seldom exist at the level required, although they have been addressed on an ad hoc basis in a variety of ways in different states and through different institutions.

DEFINING HOME CARE SERVICES

Home care is one of the major options for providing long-term care to people with functional limitations due to chronic illness or disability. The people it serves are primarily the aged and the disabled; those over 65 account for 85 to 90% of service provision (Ginzberg, Balinsky, & Ostow, 1984). It is also used as a key supportive service for families with children, though usually on a short-term basis. The goal of home care is to sustain individuals with impaired functional capacities in their own homes by providing needed personal and environmental care, supporting their own or their family's efforts to care for them. While home care includes rehabilitative elements, the term as used in this book principally refers to supportive care provided to compensate for functional limitations resulting from chronic illness. Thus, assistance with such recurring activities of daily living as dressing, ambulation, and bathing, and such basic household tasks as shopping, meal preparation, and household cleaning, is at the heart of home care as discussed herein. The concept that services are provided to compensate for specific functional limitations implies that service allocations should be based on the kind and extent of functional limitations affecting the client; however, systems for relating the one to the other are at a relatively early state in their development, as the discussions in Part II of this book will indicate.

Home care services are described by a variety of terms including homemaker, housekeeper, chore services, home attendant, personal care, and in-home supportive services, among others. The concrete services provided can be grouped into the categories of personal care, environmental care, and health-related care. Personal care includes assistance with activities of daily living such as dressing, bathing, toileting, grooming, ambulation, reminding about medications, and safety monitoring. Environmental care includes shopping, cooking, laundry, errands, and light housecleaning. Health-related services can include irrigating catheters, ostomy care, and assisting with prescribed skin care. Medically related care includes administering medicine, training in self-care, and health monitoring. These services may be supplemented by programs such as meals on wheels, friendly visiting, and telephone reassurance.

Personal care, health-related, and environmental services are provided by trained paraprofessionals working under professional supervision. Medically related home health services are provided by professionals, usually trained nurses. Supplementary services are often provided by volunteers.

This book focuses on publicly funded, nontechnical, supportive care, typically provided through agencies of state and local governments, such as departments of social services or Area Agencies on Aging, and often contracted out by such governmental agencies to nonprofit or profit-making agencies. The more technical and specialized services provided by certified home health agencies under Medicare, including skilled nursing services and home health aide services, are administered within a different framework though the content of the services and the administrative problems are often very similar.

Home care can assist in meeting the needs of the developmentally disabled and others with chronically limiting conditions who need training in self-help skills. It can also provide spouses, parents, or other family members with the assistance they need to provide personal care to a stricken relative, as well as with periodic relief and respite from continuing intensive demands. For clients, home care provides assistance with tasks that they cannot perform without help when they are living substantially on their own. Families with children may require home care because of a temporary circumstance such as the illness of a mother, or suspected or identified child abuse. Home care may also be required to provide substitute care for children or to relieve and monitor parents during stressful periods.

THE GROWTH OF HOME CARE

Perhaps the primary factor in the growing demand for home care has been expansion in the numbers of the elderly. Increases in life expectancy mean that more and more persons live to the 75-and-over age range in which functional impairment becomes common. According to the 1980 census, those 65 years of age and over numbered 25.5 million or 11.3 percent of the total U.S. population. Projections indicate that by the year 2000 there will be 31.8 million people over 65 in the United States. Among the elderly the increase in the number of people over age 75 will be especially rapid. Between 1975 and the year 2000, the 75-to-84-year-old group is expected to increase from 30 to 34 percent of all people aged 65 and older. The group aged 85 and older is expected to rise from 8 to 11% of the total elderly. In contrast, persons aged 65 to 74, less at risk for long-term care needs, are expected to decrease from 62 to 54% of the total elderly.

Because the availability or absence of natural support systems also influences the need for home care, social trends that affect family support systems increase demand for care. Increased geographic mobility means that children and other relatives may not be present to provide routine, practical assistance for the aging. Increasing participation of women in the labor force limits their availability to care for ill and aging family members, thereby cutting into the traditional supply of family caregivers. High and growing divorce rates and the resulting increase in the number of single-parent families add to the demands that compete for the attention of members of three- and four-generation families.

Policy trends also affect the demand for home care. The trend in a number of fields over the past two decades has been to move away from caring for people in institutions in favor of meeting more of their service needs in a community setting. Policies of deinstitutionalization have been pursued in such diverse fields as mental health, mental retardation, and child welfare. In the field of aging there has not so much been a policy of deinstitutionalization from nursing homes as there has been a policy to prevent or postpone institutionalization by providing community-based services such as home care. The high cost of care in nursing homes has led public officials to try to cut back on their use by limiting the expansion of nursing home beds and/or screening applicants in order to reduce inappropriate placements. More rapid discharge policies on the part of hospitals have also led to more pressure for home care. These policy thrusts have led public officials to turn increasingly to the use of home care.

Efforts to contain costs in government programs have not been limited, however, to the high-cost health services. They have also reached into home care itself as part of the general tide of fiscal constraint and as a response to a perception that the move to home care may produce hard-to-control pressures for spending. Policy actions to control the expansion and cost of home care services have been introduced in most states and localities. Home care development receives much verbal attention from public officials, but often with the expectation that home care services must be cheaper than institutional care and not an add-on to nursing home expenditures. Since nursing home care involves an inherent disincentive to care utilization that is not present with home care, expansion of home care typically does not produce net savings, and arguably should not be expected to. The argument for home care rests mostly on the more satisfactory quality of life afforded to recipients. This rationale is widely accepted in other countries (Oriol, 1985).

The impact of reduction or elimination of funding sources such as Title XX social services funds and general revenue sharing has affected the ability of states to fund home care. At the same time, demand has been increased by the pressure to minimize hospital and nursing home admissions and lengths of stay. Under the diagnostic related group (DRG) system, patients are discharged from hospitals "quicker and sicker," often directly to home care programs, which face new challenges in serving these less stable patients. Nursing home diversion efforts and changes in reimbursement rules, along with freezes in certificate-of-need approvals of nursing home stays, have resulted in a more severely disabled profile of nursing home patients than was the case in the early and mid-1970s (Hing, 1987). Increasingly, nursing homes serve the demented, the incontinent, the bedridden, and others with constant care needs. Patients with less extreme impairments but who are still quite dependent on the care of others are now less likely to be found in nursing homes, adding to pressures on home care programs which are becoming even more essential links in the long-term care system.

Thus, home care is being squeezed on one side by demographic, social, and policy trends that lead toward continuing growth in demand; and on the other side by policies aimed at keeping down public expenditures for home care itself. Home care planners and administrators must try to reconcile these pressures. One starting point for doing this is to put fiscal management practices in place that will help to ensure that the resources that become available for home care services are used as cost-effectively as possible. The following sections of this chapter offer a sense of the environment in which such management practices must operate.

FINANCING HOME CARE

There are four principal federal funding sources for home care: Medicare, Medicaid, the Social Services Block Grant (SSBG, or Title XX), and Title III of the Older Americans Act. All except Medicare are state-administered; Medicare is a direct federal program. In addition to these four major programs, there are others. For example, veterans can purchase their own home care, paid for by "aid and attendance" benefits through the Veterans Administration. Also, federal and state funds for developmental disabilities are used by state departments of mental retardation and developmental disabilities to pay for home care as an alternative to more costly institutionalization. Beyond these federal funding sources, some states and localities finance home care programs through their own tax levy appropriations. Expenditures under the four major federal programs in related depart-

**TABLE 1-1   Home Care Expenditures, 1978 and 1983
(in millions)**

Federal program	1978	1983
Medicare	$548	$1,500
Medicaid	$211	$ 597
Social Services Block Grant (Title XX)	$481	Not available
Title III, Older Americans Act	$ 17	Not available

ments, as reported by DHEW and later by DHHS, are shown in Table 1-1.

The spending variations are a function of the size and structure of the funding streams as well as the regulations governing them. The federal government no longer maintains data on the amount of home care expended under either the SSBG or the Older Americans Act, and the American Public Welfare Association also reports being unable to collect data on Title XX SSBG home care. The most recent expenditure figure available for home care under Title XX as of 1986 was $600 million for 1980 (Urban Systems Research and Engineering, 1982). State and federal Title XX expenditures were reported to have increased steadily over the last decade, at about 10 percent a year. However, Title XX has been in a state of contraction since 1980.

The National Data Base on Aging, a service of the National Association of State Units on Aging and of the Area Agencies on Aging (AAAs), collects information on a sample of Area Agencies on Aging. They report an increase from 1982 to 1984 in the percentage of home care services as a percentage of total service outlays. Housekeeping services increased from 4.5% to 7.6%, and personal care from 2.8% to 3.0%. While the sample is designed to be representative of the nation as a whole, each year's sample involves a different set of AAAs. The absolute dollar amount decreased for personal care, as did the total dollar amount for services. This may be the result of varying response rates from year to year and the use of a different set of AAAs in each sample.

Because both the Older Americans Act and the Social Services Block Grant funds are capped, the general trend has been toward open-ended Medicare and Medicaid and use of state funds and away from these capped funds. It will be helpful at this point to define each of these federal funding sources briefly, as it relates to home health care.

Medicare is an insurance program that operates as an open-ended federal program. It pays for allowable home health care services for all enrollees claiming them (when ordered by a physician and when skilled nursing care is required). In practice, the allowable services are short-term and transitional in nature. The Medicare home health program is limited to people who have suffered acute health episodes and require skilled nursing care, and new limitations were administratively imposed in 1985 (Leader, 1986). Services can be provided by certified home health agencies that are reimbursed through fiscal intermediaries. (Fiscal management relating to these services is not directly covered in this publication.)

Medicaid serves only the indigent, including those who have become so because they have "spent down" their assets and income for medical care, to a level typically well below the poverty line. Medicaid, too, is an open-ended program, at least in the sense that the federal government sets no limits on the amount of its payment to states for programs serving eligible recipients. However, Medicaid is not a federally administered program; rather, it is funded on the basis of a formula that matches state and/or local expenditures with federal funds. Because of the matching requirement, the resources available are limited by the capacity or willingness of a state or its localities to pay their share, as much as half of the total. Because only certain services and populations are federally mandated to be included by states that participate in the program, coverage varies by state for optional services and for populations other than those eligible for Aid for Dependent Children (AFDC) or Supplemental Security Income (SSI). At present, the only home care service that states are required to provide under Medicaid is home health care, which can only be provided through certified home health agencies under orders of a physician and with nursing supervision. Personal care services, provided under physician orders and characterized by a lower level of nursing supervision, are available as a Medicaid optional service or through waivers. The 1981 Omnibus Budget Reconciliation Act allowed state Medicaid agencies to provide coverage of "home and community-based services" to persons at risk of nursing home placement under a Section 2176 waiver. By March 1985, 46 states received Section 2176 waivers for one or more target populations (Burwell, 1986); some of these covered only limited geographical areas within a state.

States have often set lower reimbursement rates for Medicaid home health care than for Medicare. This has served as a disincentive for providers to participate in home health aide services under Medicaid. The role of the Medicaid program in financing home care in a particular state depends on such factors as (1) the number of services covered; (2) the strictness of the income eligibility test (e.g., whether people who are not on AFDC or SSI but are on Medicaid are included and whether people are allowed to "spend down" to the medical need level); and (3) the provider reimbursement rates set by the state. Rates of reimbursement as well as the size of the service population influence how attractive participation in the program is to providers.

The *Social Services Block Grant* (Title XX of the Social Security Act) and *Title III of the Older Americans Act* (OAA) involve aid to states by the federal government in accordance with specific annual appropriations. These resources are not automatically applied to home care. The type of services funded under these two programs and the amount of resources allocated to them are determined by priorities established in state and local planning processes. Home care services funded under the Social Services Block Grant are in many states primarily environmental, with some personal care allowed as long as it is subsidiary to social services. SSBG eligibility is not limited by age but is means tested. States have some latitude in setting the level of income eligibility and may set sliding fee scales. States are no longer required to match SSBG funds. Older Americans Act services, by definition, are limited to the elderly (aged 60 and up) and have no income test. States are required to match federal funds under Title III, paying 10 percent of service and 25 percent of administrative costs.

The diverse roles played by states and localities in allocating resources and in determining eligibility for home care services make it difficult to generalize about the relative importance of the different funding sources across the country. Expenditure data do, however, show that Medicare is the largest federal program, while the Older Americans Act program is the smallest. SSBG and Medicaid are the primary sources of funding for state and locally administered long-term home care, but comparison of the dollars contributed to home care by SSBG funds and Medicaid is not possible for recent years because no national data are currently available on what fraction of SSBG dollars is spent on home care. Which of the two programs predominates in a given state is largely a result of the configuration of the two programs in the state. This tends to be a function of the financial commitment the state makes to the two programs and of the income standards and services available under them. As an entitlement program, Medicaid has different implications for state and local planning than either SSBG or OAA programs, because anyone who is eligible for service is entitled to receive it. Therefore, controlling budgetary growth is an issue that is more problematic in Medicaid than it is in the fixed-budget SSBG and OAA programs, though it is problematic there as well. As a result, most states have adopted quite restrictive limits on the availability of Medicaid funds for home care, fearing that more flexible standards under an open-ended entitlement program could lead to runaway expansion of program costs.

ORGANIZATIONAL STRUCTURE

It is even more difficult to generalize about how home care programs are organized across the country than it is to generalize about the relative contributions of the different federal funding sources. Whether the state agency designated to administer one of the principal federal programs administers it directly or in conjunction with local agencies depends on the relationships between state and local government in each state. Furthermore, the decision as to whether Social Services Block Grant, Medicaid, and Older Americans Act programs are administered by the same or different state or local agencies depends on the nature of the state and local structure. The decision as to whether home care services are delivered directly by public agencies or contracted out also depends on state and local policies.

Agencies at the state level involved in the administration of publicly funded home care services typically include the offices responsible for Medicaid (typically either the state health department or the state public welfare agency); those responsible for the Social Services Block Grant (typically the state public welfare agency); and those responsible for services to the aged (typically the state office on aging). A review of reported organizational structures as of the early 1980s indicates that in 20 states all these functions were responsibilities of a single human services superagency. Often, however, they report separately to the governor, raising significant problems of coordination for home care (American Public Welfare Association, 1982). In 28 states, Older Americans Act services were administered in a separate state agency from social services and Medicaid. In several states, including some of these 28, social services and Medicaid are themselves in separate agencies.

To complicate the picture further, some states administer social services and Medicaid directly, while others supervise their administration by counties or other political subdivisions. In 1982, 27 states fell into the first category and 22 into the second. One state had a mixed pattern. Further, Older Americans Act programs are generally administered by Area Agencies on Aging, which may be part of the local government structure or may be nonprofit agencies.

In addition to the variations in the organizational structure of the agencies administering home care, there are variations in the approaches that these agencies have adopted in performing the two major programmatic functions—case management and service delivery. Case management can be handled in at least three ways: It can be performed by the administering agency's own casework staff, independent of the service provision functions; it can be performed in whole or part by a service-providing agency as part of its contracted service management role; or it can be performed by an agency under contract to provide case management services, which, in turn, arranges for the provision of home care by other providers. How these functions are performed has implications for staffing and employment relationships, described in Chapters 4 and 5. These relationships have considerable fiscal implications for administrators.

Public agencies employ three major strategies for delivering the actual direct home care services. One strategy is to provide services directly, using staff that is hired, trained, and supervised by the public agency itself. Another approach is for a public agency to contract with other public, nonprofit, or proprietary agencies to deliver services to the agency's clients. A third approach is for the public agency to pay the home care client to employ an individual to provide the needed services to the client. There can be a variety of patterns within a single state. Of the 21 states that provided descriptions of their home care programs to the Home Care Fiscal Management Project in response to an initial request for information about their management

TABLE 1-2 Program Models

Case management variations	Service delivery variations
Direct provision	Direct provision
Contracted to service delivery agency	Contracted to service delivery agency
Contracted to case management agency	Self-employed individual

practices, 19 contracted for services with provider agencies. But eight of these states also provided services through arrangements with self-employed individuals. In three states some services were provided directly. One state provided all services directly. Decisions about which staffing patterns to use are often driven by the labor costs of the home care workers—the major home care expense.

As can be seen, it is difficult within this range of variations to identify anything that comes close to being a norm in the organization of home care. Table 1-2 and Figure 1-1 depict the basic system options in home care. Table 1-2 lists the major variations in the ways that case management and service delivery functions are handled. Figure 1-1 shows the two major alternative approaches to administrative structure; that is, it shows how federal funding from a particular source can go to a designated state agency, which either itself performs or administers case management and service delivery functions or delegates their adminis-

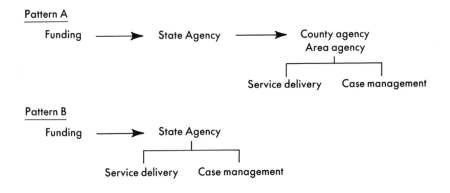

FIGURE 1-1 Funding models.

tration to local agencies. Most commonly, the administrative and organizational functions under each federal program are performed independently of those of the other home care financing sources; exceptions to this may occur where two or more programs are under the umbrella of the same agency. Exceptions also occur where states have tried to deal with the problem of fragmentation through interagency agreements or by placing two or more funding sources in a single administrative unit. For example, Georgia, Oregon, and South Dakota each have integrated their three state-administered programs into a single framework. With respect to case management, the norm appears to be for the administering agency to retain most of the case management functions. In contrast, service delivery appears to be contracted out in most instances.

PROBLEMS IN FISCAL MANAGEMENT

Given the multiplicity of funding sources and organizational arrangements that shape the structure of home care, it is not surprising that problems arise as administrators and planners seek to further the development of home care services and yet keep program costs under control. Two key issues related to administering home care programs are: first, how to fund expansion and development of services and, second, how to make existing funds go farther.

The first issue—how to fund expansion and development of home care—has become of greater significance as the federal government has capped expenditures and set restrictions on provider rates or client services. Short of convincing the state legislature to increase the home care budget, there are few options for administrators except to learn to live within these limitations.

There have been a number of time-limited Medicare waiver demonstrations to test the cost effectiveness of broadening the range and eligibility of home health services. Some states have instituted programs that pay subsidies to families caring for ill members. Some have sought to expand their home care services by tapping open-ended Medicaid personal care services and most recently by applying for Medicaid waivers that broaden either the scope of services permitted or client eligibility or both. The requirement under Medicaid for statewide coverage can also be waived, encouraging states to demonstrate cost effectiveness of a broader range of services on a small scale before attempting to go statewide. Time-limited Section 2176 community care waivers have enabled state Medicaid agencies to begin to develop long-term care programs, especially for personal care services. According to the federal rules for the waivers, none of these programs is supposed to cost the state more Medicaid dollars than would have been spent without the waiver, and all are limited to Medicaid recipients who might otherwise require nursing home care.

The issue of how to make existing funds go farther, or at least to ensure that they are being spent in a cost-effective manner, is at base a question concerning the efficient management of program dollars. In this regard, some of the most frequent questions that arise are as follows:

1. *Allocation and targeting of resources.* Are service hours being awarded uniformly and fairly? What objective methods are there for targeting those most in need of services? Are there any formulas that can help allocate staff and dollars among localities or counties within a state? Are other sources of funding being tapped or leveraged? Do case management systems serve as effective gatekeepers and help control costs? What practices might help achieve both reasonable service costs and safe and effective care?

2. *Program integration.* Are there ways to integrate the various funding streams at the administrative and/or provider level so as to reduce program fragmentation across the different programs? Can computers help keep track of funding streams and assist in billing each source?

3. *Determination of costs and rate setting.* What are the actual costs of a program? What should the unit of service be? How stable are costs over time, and can they be forecast? Are case management and training direct or indirect costs? What cost centers should be used, and what should they include? How should rates be set for contracts—by line item or by unit cost? Should they be fixed or adjusted for cost? Can costs of different types of service, types of providers, or various localities and states be compared? What costs and benefits are associated with different service delivery systems?

4. *Cash flow.* Are there mechanisms that public agencies

can use to advance funds for agencies, particularly for salaries? How should settlements be handled if there are overpayments?

5. *Monitoring fiscal and service performance.* What administrative and fiscal controls can be used to assure that
clients are receiving authorized services and that payments
are made to providers only for what is authorized? What
performance indicators are there for evaluating and monitoring contractor performance? What controls or sanctions over providers should be put in place? What use
should be made of post-audit information? What practices
can help control contract costs? Are there any valid and
reliable methods for measuring outcomes? Can various systems link their service and fiscal data?

6. *Management information and fiscal control systems.*
Are there readily adaptable information systems that can
provide service, cost, and expenditure data in a timely
fashion to assist in budget forecasting and policy planning?
How can computers effectively be used to support program management? How can state Medicaid and other
large data bases be used more effectively? How can such
information systems handle the complexities of cost sharing and ''spend-down'' requirements?

INNOVATIVE PRACTICES IN HOME CARE

The chapters in Part II of this book describe in detail five innovative programs and their practices. The following paragraphs offer brief descriptions of how these members of the Home Care
Fiscal Management Consortium have dealt with some of the preceding six fiscal issues in their programs.

Alameda County

Concern that home care hours and, as a result, service dollars
were being awarded to clients in a way that achieved inequitable
results led Alameda County in California to redesign the assessment and hour-award process in its In-Home Supportive Services program, financed under the Social Services Block Grant. A
unique aspect of Alameda County's effort to standardize assess-

ment and award decisions is the introduction of microcomputers into the process. The computer guides social workers in their service award decisions by providing them with instant information on the service hours awarded to clients with similar characteristics. The introduction of this computer-assisted service award process has resulted in more consistent service-hour allocations across the caseload, thereby improving the fairness of service-dollar allocations.

In addition to improving the fairness of client service awards, Alameda's redesigned system has other features that assist program managers and administrators. The system computes an eligibility index for each client which provides an objective measure of the client's functional capacities. This index is used to set the threshold of eligibility of services and is one element managers use for budget control and forecasting expenditures. The computerized award records are used to generate periodic reports on the consistency of award decisions, thus facilitating monitoring of performance of this key program function. Also, the system provides a computerized data base on the current caseload, which, when linked with fiscal data by a budget analysis program, has enhanced Alameda County's planning and budget forecasting capacity.

Connecticut

The Connecticut Department on Aging's Promotion of Independent Living program has adopted a comprehensive case management model that seeks to assure that clients are allocated the most appropriate mix of services, regardless of funding source of those services. The program also has the objective of extending the department's budgeted capacity to purchase services for clients by coordinating and leveraging other public, private, community, and family resources through the mechanism of case management. A distinguishing feature of Connecticut's program is that the state contracts with private nonprofit agencies to serve as entry points for clients coming into the program. The agencies provide case management services for eligible clients on a statewide basis. In order to hold the contractor accountable for its case management services and for using the department's own service dollars only when other sources are not available, the Department on Aging has adopted a "performance-based contracting" system. Under the terms of the contract, the department receives a regular series of reports from the case management agency which allow it to monitor such things as case activity, leveraging of outside resources, commitment of program service dollars, and client costs with and without leveraged resources. Contract payments to the nonprofit case manager are tied to satisfactory performance. Use of such a performance contract enables Connecticut to retain control of program resources and to ensure that its policy of optimizing its own service dollars is being followed. The program design enables the Connecticut Department on Aging to mobilize the full range of available funding sources, not simply its own, on behalf of its clients, thereby integrating various home care services at the client level.

Texas

As part of an effort to improve the quality and quantity of home care services across the state, the Texas Department of Human Services reviewed its contracting practices and developed contract procedures that increased state control over the cost and quality of service in both its Medicaid and Social Services Block Grant programs. Texas contracts with home care providers to deliver service for a flat rate, which is developed on the basis of state analysis of provider cost reports. The rates are statewide in the Title XIX program and by contract in the SSBG program. The contracts also include contractor service performance requirements, such as timely initiation of service, which form the basis of monitoring provider service delivery. There are established sanctions in the SSBG program, and penalties are also planned for the Title XIX program for failure to comply with contract requirements. To facilitate fiscal and service audits, the department developed three documents: the client authorization, a worker timesheet that includes the client's plan of care, and billing forms. Together, these forms provide an audit trail linking fiscal and service information. Since these forms were introduced, audit exceptions have decreased. Texas's contract system has also eliminated confusion among providers about performance expectations. Another feature of Texas's home care program is that the case management for its Medicaid and SSBG programs are integrated into a single operation.

Washington

In the state of Washington, the Bureau of Aging and Adult Services has sought to maximize use of its program resources and fiscal control of its Chore Services program through the contracting process. While the contracting responsibility is delegated to Area Agencies on Aging, the bureau has stipulated that the contracts must be awarded competitively and that reimbursement must be on a fixed unit-rate basis. In this way the state tries to maximize the service units that the Chore Services program (funded from SSBG and State General Fund revenues) can purchase. Washington credits its contracting practice with stabilizing service costs. Without cost adjustments, providers have an incentive to avoid losses and possibly achieve a small surplus. However, to control against providers' gaining cost efficiencies at the expense of service to the client, Washington, like Connecticut and Texas, uses a performance-based contract, tying reimbursement to satisfactory service performance, not simply the fact of having delivered a service. The combination of its rate-setting method and its performance controls has, in Washington's experience, shifted the focus of fiscal control away from the details of provider costs and onto the content of the service unit.

New York City

When New York City moved to contract out its Home Attendant Program (funded under Medicaid as a personal care service), it chose a different reimbursement method from either Texas or Washington. While lacking cost history for "vendorized" service provision, New York City wanted to achieve strict control over provider costs and also wanted to find a way to solve the cash flow problems of the small community-based agencies that were among its providers. As a result, it elected to reimburse providers for costs on a strict line-item basis, based on administrative guidelines that specify staffing and salary levels and allowable amounts for office space, equipment, and other overhead components. In addition, administrative payments were split off from payments for direct-service costs, creating a two-tiered payment stream, in order to guarantee that direct-service payments would not be held up and threaten service continuity. Thus, providers were advanced a portion of direct-service funds, based on the hours of care they had been authorized to deliver, plus a monthly administrative advance. These advances guaranteed cash flow for the providers while they allowed New York to have strict cost-based reimbursement and to foster the development of small providers who lacked the capital needed to cover start-up costs. This system provided data that enabled the city to begin to move to a unit rate.

Common Themes

A number of other states and localities, as well as the consortium members, have also tackled the major issues of concern to home care administrators. All of these efforts have revealed important common themes. One recurrent theme is the need to create a contractual framework that allows the government agencies that fund and supervise the programs, and the provider agencies that actually deliver the services, to perform their respective roles most appropriately. This includes providing accountability by provider agencies, incorporating incentives for cost control on the part of those agenicies, and assuring both the flow of needed financial and programmatic information and the exercise of appropriate dimensions of control in the contractual relationship. Models of the contractual relationship described in Part II vary along a strong-control/weak-control continuum and represent alternative solutions to the problem of how to purchase service at the lowest possible cost while assuring that service quality is maintained. (Since service quality is difficult to measure directly, the quality-assurance consideration usually involves assurance of key service inputs.)

Another recurring theme in home care management involves the search for more satisfactory methods and procedures with which to assess the need for home care services and determine the number of hours of care per week or month to be provided. Assessment and case management methods vary widely and have been developed locally after considerable effort. Connecticut, with its case management system, and Alameda County, with the microcomputer-based equity system, represent significant though varying models for addressing the assessment and service assignment problem. The Alameda County system also presents approaches to integrated management and utilization of the data both on client characteristics and needs and on program budgeting and financial management.

The theme of integrated information management turned out to be a central one in our investigation of home care management practices. Of particular importance were the integration of various financially related functions with one another and the combination of financial information with data usually considered "programmatic," such as client impairments. What many of the more promising approaches to home care administration seemed to have in common was a management process that combined types of information and functions that often are managed elsewhere in a segregated fashion. Integration of the basic functions of *budgeting, accounting, performance measurement,* and *auditing* was a particular focus. These functions, in turn, support the three basic management processes of *decision making, implementation,* and *assessment.* These functions and processes are the subject of the next chapter.

Understanding of these innovations in the areas of contractual arrangements, assessment of need, and integration of financial data with program functions is an important key to a healthier and more effective home care system.

2

Fiscal Management: Governmental and Home Care Applications

Integration of management functions generally, and integrated fiscal management in particular, has been difficult to achieve for many public agencies administering home care programs. Several difficulties present themselves. Many home care programs are still in the early stages of administrative evolution and often lack the infrastructure of information management systems, sophisticated accounting procedures, computers, and other tools that facilitate integrated management. The diversity of funding sources, and their very different reporting and eligibility requirements, complicate the task. Concepts of integrated financial management that originally developed with respect to general financial functions of state and local government are not always easy to adapt to the more specialized field of home care management. Nevertheless, it seems appropriate in this chapter to place home care fiscal management issues in the context of broader questions of public financial management. Public administrators in home care frequently express the need to link service and fiscal data, and they ask for assistance with this goal.

Since the mid-1970s, the level of interest in improved fiscal management has been high in state and local governments. Fiscal crises have highlighted the need for better and more accurate fiscal systems. Pressures from lending institutions, bond rating organizations, business firms, the federal government, and the public for greater governmental accountability and financial control have generated strong interest in such improvements.

Despite these developments, the state of fiscal management practices at the state and local level has remained mixed at best. For example, few states and even fewer localities have implemented accounting systems that follow generally accepted accounting principles as defined for governments by such groups as the Municipal Finance Officers' Association. Few state or local governments have adopted performance management systems—known as management-by-objectives systems—that include indicators of service delivery and systematically compare actual accomplishments against preestablished plans or targets for quality and quantity of service delivery. While most governments have a financial auditing process, few have implemented modern management or performance auditing systems.

What is true of fiscal management of general governmental functions is even more true of publicly administered home care programs. Most home care agencies operate under severe constraints of administrative costs and staffing which limit the sophistication of the systems they can implement. Management information and control are even more difficult because the services are provided in an unusually decentralized and diverse manner. There is no central service site where direct-service workers perform their functions, as there is in institutional operations. Services are provided, in most instances, not directly by government employees but by employees of private nonprofit or proprietary agencies or even by individual "independent contractors." Provider agencies often have complex structures of their own, sometimes involving multiple corporate entities. Mixing different funding streams adds further complexity. Thus, the challenge to public administrators of home care as well as to provider agencies is great.

As the examples in Part II of this book show, some local and state jurisdictions have developed their own innovative approaches to the challenges of financial management. Even as these are developed, however, the broader challenge of systematic improvements remains. To help meet this challenge, it is important for home care administrators to consider how to integrate the various components of their fiscal management systems into a balanced whole.

COMPONENTS OF A FISCAL MANAGEMENT SYSTEM

Fiscal management in a governmental setting involves the following basic functions:

1. *Budgeting*—the process of preparing and carrying out the fiscal plan that involves balancing anticipated expenditures with available revenues
2. *Accounting*—the basic fiscal record-keeping and expenditure-control tool
3. *Performance Measurement*—establishing and monitoring targets for agency performance and service delivery
4. *Auditing*—the process of evaluating financial and service operations that provides vital feedback that can then be used to strengthen budgeting, management, and control

These four functions are the heart of the planning, management, and control systems through which state and local governments and their agencies decide what they want to do and make sure that their decisions are carried out or modified to reflect changing conditions. These four management functions support the following three basic processes, which usually occur in the sequence presented:

1. *Decision Making.* This is the process of planning and analysis in which the central activity is budgeting. This is where decisions are made about what services government will provide, how much they will cost, in what quantity they will be provided, and where the money will come from.
2. *Implementation.* This is the process of management and control of governmental operations in which the central activities are accounting and performance measurement. Accounting provides for monitoring of actual spending so that management knows if it is sticking to its budget plan. Performance measurement provides a report on the actual operations of government so that officials know if they are

meeting their service delivery targets.
3. *Assessment.* This is the process of evaluation and feedback of which the central activity is auditing. Assessment comes after the fact to tell state and local governments whether results conformed to their plan. These functions are best met by two types of audit—financial and performance. Both are necessary for full-scale evaluation.

These four basic functions of budgeting, accounting, performance measurement, and auditing will be discussed here, together with a review of the benefits of linking the four functions to one another to achieve more effective approaches to control, management, and planning (Hayes, Grossman, Thomas, & Mechling, 1982).

Budgeting

The budget is a vital element in decision making, often *the* central element. The budget is the plan of a government or an agency for allocating its resources among competing demands.

In most state and local governments, the annual budget is initially prepared on the basis of requests for funds from operating units or agencies of the government. These requests are reviewed, adjusted, and merged into a single document by the chief executive, who submits the proposed budget for review, change, and approval by the legislature. The departments and other operating units of government are then responsible for administering the adopted budget within the limits set by the legislature. This pattern of submission of requests, executive budget formulation, legislative adoption, and executive administration holds true today for most governmental units, despite a vast array of approaches to budgeting.

While states and localities put their budgets together in many different ways, there are primarily two types of budgets—operating and capital. Typically, the operating budget pays for annually recurring expenses, such as salaries of public employees, supplies, rent, and the cost of contracted services. The capital budget pays for the cost of constructing buildings and purchasing major pieces of equipment such as trucks.

Schick (1966) has divided budgeting into three key aspects: control, management, and planning. Each of these functions corresponds to an important feature of governance.

The origins of public budgeting were connected with the *control* concept, that is, the need to assure that appropriations are spent for the purpose intended by the legislature in its approval of the budget. In its simplest sense, this requirement means that, if money is appropriated for a home attendant's salary, then that is what it must be used for and not for anything else. Furthermore, only the specific amount designated for the attendant's salary can be so used. The introduction of the control concept as the basis of the budget process has led to the "line-item" approach to budgeting. Each proposed item of expenditure is to be listed in as much detail as possible so that a careful record can be maintained to control spending and limit it to legitimate items. Under the line-item approach, budgets become detailed lists of proposed items of expenditure, with the amount of each employee's salary and each item of supply or equipment listed separately so that as spending occurs it can be checked off against an approved appropriation.

Once the effort to control the details of public expenditure had succeeded, the attention of people concerned with improving state and local government finance began to shift to issues of *management* and *performance.* Performance budgeting embodies a management-oriented approach to the budget. Its principal thrust has been to determine how government services can be most efficiently provided. The work of the government is seen in terms of activities and tasks and of the organizational units performing them. Budget categories are cast in functional terms such as "home care services," rather than as separate line items or objects of expenditure.

The *planning* approach to budgeting is a more recent orientation. It emphasizes neither fiscal control nor operational efficiency but, rather, the rational resolution of policy choices in both expenditure and revenue raising. In this model, government operations are perceived primarily in terms of their purposes or objectives and the budget is organized by programs defined by the objectives they serve, rather than by objects of functional activities. An example of such a definition would be to set an objective for providing long-term care, with home care viewed as one option for achieving the goal. This approach to budgeting seeks to focus attention on the cost-effectiveness of a program in comparison with alternative means of achieving the same objective.

In practice, of course, these theoretically distinct approaches to budgeting overlap. The broad purpose-defined program of the planning-oriented budget can be subdivided into the activities and tasks of the management budget. Program analysis for the planning-oriented budget must also contend with the same issues of operational efficiency with which the management-oriented budget is primarily concerned.

A modern budget system must serve all three purposes: control, management, and planning. This is not easy, because a different organization of information is best suited for each purpose. The structure of the budget, in turn, determines to some degree how budget decisions are made. The line-item budget directs attention to the material and the personal services to be financed. A management-oriented budget structured by organizational units focuses on the amounts necessary to support the various departments and agencies of government. The program or planning budget looks at spending proposals in terms of the services they are intended to provide to citizens. The need for budget systems to serve *all* of these functions effectively has involved a progressive increase in the demands placed by budgeting on the other three fiscal management processes of accounting, auditing, and performance measurement.

To date, more emphasis has been placed by home care administrators on control functions than on management or planning. This has been in recognition of the critical importance, especially for agencies limited to SSBG and OAA funding, as many are, of keeping spending within strict limits. The New York City case in Chapter 10 is an illustration of a primarily control-oriented approach. Management orientation has begun to appear, also. Washington State's unit-rate contracting is a good illustration of the use of a performance, or management, approach. To date, no full-scale example of a planning approach to budgeting for home care has been identified; however, Alameda County's computerized assessment system has proven surprisingly adaptable to evaluating alternative policy scenarios, a key step in planning.

Accounting

Accounting serves three basic purposes: budgetary control, accountability and internal control, and information. Accounting is the basic element of the budgetary control structure. It is the means by which commitments and expenditures of public funds are limited to the amounts and purposes authorized in the budget. Limitations on spending are set by (1) the amounts provided in the budget as enacted by the legislative body and (2) any budget modifications approved over the course of the year. In home care programs, limits can also be set in other ways, such as in the form of legislative ''caps'' on spending. Conceptually, the implementation of accounting controls to enforce budgetary limits on expenditures or obligations is a relatively straightforward matter. The amount available for expenditure in any account is specified by the appropriation or other legislative authorization, as modified by budgetary allocation or apportionment. When the balance available is inadequate to cover a proposed expenditure, the accounting department usually returns the voucher to the agency with a statement indicating that sufficient funds are not available. The performance of the budgetary control function must be both effective and prompt. To accomplish this, controls must be implemented at a level that is not so detailed as to impede the expeditious processing of transactions.

The accounting system also incorporates the accountability and internal control procedures by which financial commitments are made and reviewed. These include the assignment of responsibility and accountability and the operation of internal controls necessary to assure the integrity of the system. Effective internal control depends, first, on a clear-cut assignment of authority and responsibility to specific officials for spending decisions and the custody of resources. Another element of internal control consists of procedures and regulations governing the commitment, disbursement, and receipt of funds and the acquisition, custody, and disposition of other assets. Such procedures and regulations establish standards for the documentation of transactions for higher-level approval and for allocating responsibility for certain functions. A third element of control includes the various means of assuring that the safeguards incorporated in procedures and regulations are effectively implemented. This is a major concern of the independent audit, which should include the review of a sample of individual transactions, reconciliation of bank balances, and other measures such as edits in the payment process.

The reporting of financial information is required to meet the needs of a variety of users, both within and outside government. The character of the data needed varies among the different users and purposes. Meeting all of these needs may require a capacity to aggregate and report data at several different points in the transaction sequence and under several alternative structures, rather than just a single chart of accounts.

Local and state governments administering home care programs need sound internal accounting systems to support and control their expenditure efforts. In addition, those governments that provide services via contracts with voluntary or proprietary agencies need to promulgate and enforce sound accounting and reporting standards for their contractors. Some approaches to this process are discussed in Part II. For example, the Texas program appears to be among the nation's more advanced in its integrated approach to accounting; the Connecticut program makes use of a central nonprofit contractor to coordinate its information flows; and in New York City heavy reliance on community-based nonprofits to deliver services has created an especially acute need for reliable and simplified accounting approaches.

Performance Measurement

Management and performance accountability are not usually discussed as basic fiscal management functions, yet a system or budget decision making and expenditure control cannot be truly meaningful unless it helps to make sure that the local government gets its money's worth in goods and services from its expenditures.

Performance measurement is the means by which a government introduces into its fiscal management practices a system of monitor the efficiency and the effectiveness of the services it provides. A performance measurement system provides better and more systematic information on the goods and services produced by government agencies than is otherwise available. With this information the heads of operating agencies, central agency managers, and elected officials can more easily answer questions such as, How well are we doing? or, What can we do to provide better services? To answer these questions requires being able to identify the strengths and shortcomings in current performance and to make choices based on this information.

Performance reporting and accountability are basic ingredients of modern budget decision making and effective program management. Without performance data, program and issue analysis in the budget process is nearly impossible. Without performance accountability, there is no assurance that management will actually achieve the performance level supported by the budget.

Inherent in the concept of performance measurement are three component elements:

- Goals to be achieved
- Measures and targets to be used to monitor progress in reaching goals
- Periodic reports on progress

Goals are statements of purpose and direction toward which public resources of the government or a particular public agency are to be guided. For example, a program goal for a department of human resources might be to increase the availability of alternative means of providing long-term care to the elderly at the lowest feasible cost. Home care and nursing homes would be among the major options to be considered in achieving such a goal.

Measures and targets are more specific and quantifiable than goals. They can be used to monitor actual results and to assess performance against targets. Three major performance characteristics can be used in target setting and in measuring and monitoring governmental performance:

1. *Efficiency*. This measures performance in the use of resources. Efficiency is not measured directly; rather, it is the ratio of output to input. In home care a typical efficiency measure might compare the average cost of providing one hour of service to a homebound client under two different provider arrangements.
2. *Quality of Service*. This assesses variations in the characteristics of service that are not reflected in quantitative measures of output. Some of the attributes of service quality that can be described include timeliness, responsiveness, thoroughness, accuracy, and courtesy. The time it takes to initiate service to a client, starting with the date of referral, is an example of a possible measure of timeliness for a home care agency.
3. *Program Effectiveness*. This measures progress toward achieving goals. It is almost always more difficult to mea-

sure program effectiveness or impact than it is to measure program efficiency. Program effectiveness can be measured by comparing observed results to one or more of the following: a similar target population not served by the program, the situation before the program began, some ideal situation such as absence of poverty or malnutrition, or an administratively established goal. In home care, for example, a program-impact measure might compare the percentage of clients who receive chore services and who remain in their homes after a given time period with the status of a control group of nonaccepted applicants who were otherwise eligible and who did not receive this service.

Periodic progress reports on performance criteria summarize accomplishments and explain which objectives were achieved, which were not, and the reasons for the shortfalls. The two most common types of reporting techniques are (1) comparison of current performance levels against a plan or target and (2) measurement of progress against a sequential schedule of major events or "milestones."

A performance measurement system can also be viewed as a form of contract between top management and key program managers. Funds are included in the budget for each program on the premise that performance will meet agreed-upon targets. Performance measurement improves the linkages between financial decisions and expected results and increases the accountability of program managers in achieving planned results.

In the home care field, as in many other aspects of public administration, performance measurement tends to be the least well developed of the four basic systems of fiscal management. Three of the major case studies presented in Part II do, however, deal with some of its aspects:

- Connecticut uses a performance-based contract between the Department on Aging and a statewide case management contractor. This arrangement provides monthly measures of performance against preestablished goals for both service and expenditure levels.
- The Texas system relies on an integrated fiscal and performance measurement system as the core of its approach to documentation, control, and monitoring.

- Alameda County's approach emphasizes performance measures in one aspect of its home care system—feedback on service levels—so as to enable workers to make more equitable decisions.

In coming years it will be important for more home care agencies to adopt and adapt such systems so that they can assure their funding sources of effective and efficient program information and control.

Auditing

The three components of fiscal management discussed in the preceding sections include all of the elements basic to the internal functioning of an organization. What accounting, budgeting, and performance measurement do not provide, however, is an independent assessment of operations. This can be established only by an after-the-fact review and evaluation performed by organizations and individuals independent of those responsible for the activities that are evaluated. The audit is the established form for such an evaluation.

The most basic and essential type of audit is the annual financial and compliance audit conducted according to generally accepted auditing standards of the American Institute of Certified Public Accountants. This type of audit assesses the integrity of the functioning of a fiscal management system. It includes a review of whether financial reports fairly reflect the fiscal position of the government or agency under generally accepted accounting principles, whether the safeguards against unauthorized expenditures are adequate, whether required procedures are consistently followed, and whether cost and performance are accurately reported.

A second type of audit examines program results. For all practical purposes the program-results audit is a form of evaluation. Its objective is to determine the extent to which programs and operations achieve their intended results. An example of such an audit is one that looks to see whether an increase in home care had any impact on nursing home utilization rates or whether an elderly person's self-perception was strengthened by participation in a senior citizens program. Program audits can also examine whether there are alternative solutions that might yield desired results at a lower cost.

The economy and efficiency audit is the third element in the concept of the comprehensive audit as developed by the United States General Accounting Office, the public sector leader in its field. Also known as a management or performance audit, review of this character is concerned with the quality of management structure and organizational as well as operational performance. It identifies the extent and apparent causes of inefficiencies, failures to achieve management objectives, and deviations from managerial policies. At its completion, recommendations are made for corrective action.

Audits and evaluations constitute the feedback loop in the fiscal system. They provide the periodic checkups necessary to assure that the system is functioning satisfactorily and to identify areas for correction. Some audits, particularly financial and compliance audits, must be done by licensed or certified public accountants independent of the audited organization. Other audits, such as a management or program results audit, can also be done internally by organizations or individuals with accounting credentials.

Home care administrators are accustomed to the use of financial audits in assuring that public funds allocated to provider agencies are properly accounted for. Of the examples presented in Part II, the Washington situation is especially relevant in this regard. This state uses the auditing process not to recapture any profit or surplus but rather to inform the budgeting process in coming years; this is an imaginative use of the feedback aspect of the audit. In addition, Washington uses audits to test contractor accounting and internal controls, to check on the legality of expenditures, and to assure that federal and state regulations are observed. Texas changed to a unit-rate approach instead of cost reimbursement as a result of information learned from audits. Except for these instances, however, it seems that most uses of audit in home care involve its more traditional aspects of assurance of fiscal probity and compliance with regulations. The concept of program results or management audits, as described in this section, do not yet appear to have been much developed or applied in the field.

THE BENEFITS OF INTEGRATION

Most existing fiscal information systems evolved from rather independent beginnings within the individual financial functions. Accountants set up systems to meet formal reporting requirements; budgeting people establish systems for budget planning and control; and operating managers set up their own systems to measure performance. At the outset, definitions and files are usually not consistent from one system to another and, for most purposes, do not need to be. While each system measures a dimension of organizational performance, they do so from differing perspectives.

In most governmental applications today, fiscal functions such as payroll, accounting, budgeting, and purchasing are still handled by independent information systems. Each of these systems has its own data entry and processing routines. Data from one function are not used as automated inputs to another. Indeed, transaction items applicable to various reporting systems are generally posted as separate manual tasks.

In integrated systems, fiscal data (and sometimes performance data as well) are consolidated into a unified data base that can meet the service needs of many separate agency functions. When successfully accomplished, an integrated approach to data entry avoids duplication in the recording and processing of data and also provides for timely analysis and control.

The first step toward integration is often to tie together the basic accounting and budgeting functions. This makes certain that budgeting and accounting can use each other's data and identifies cost and responsibility centers for management control. This initial level of integration typically extends to the payroll system as well as to other data files on entities involved in financial transactions such as personnel files, vendor files, and tax files.

Performance data are rarely collected as a by-product of financial record keeping, and in fact performance audit usually requires that special new procedures be established. As a result, performance information systems are often independent of the financial information system, although they often adopt the same organizational and budgetary structure.

Integrated systems are a working reality in an increasing number of state and local governments. The benefits from an integrated system consist for the most part of greatly increased opportunities for better decision making, more effective control of both expenditures and performance, and improved program management. Integrated fiscal management systems impose the discipline of accountability on finances and also on program performance. Budget allocations can be coupled with data on performance targets that involve program output, quality, efficiency, and effectiveness. This introduces a capacity for managerial control and informed decision making that can make the job of delivering high-quality service at a reasonable cost more manageable.

In addition, there are often more concrete, dollars-and-cents benefits. The best example is in the claiming of costs under federal programs. Many governments do not have financial information systems that permit them to determine accurately the indirect costs associated with grant-assisted projects or programs such as Medicaid. As a result, these costs are often underclaimed. In governments with large federal grant programs, the increase in reimbursements resulting from a new financial information system will often be enough to amortize the cost of the information system in a brief period of time.

On balance, an integrated system is desirable both from the viewpoint of dollars and cents and from that of more responsive management. It offers to state and local governments a major opportunity to link fiscal management functions together and to improve planning and analysis. What is true for government as a whole seems also likely to prove true with respect to home care programs. Agencies often feel that their day-to-day needs in fiscal management are so pressing that full-scale system integration is a luxury they can't afford. This may be an understandable reaction, but it is also apt to be a short-sighted one. Integration can be taken as a goal to build toward; it need not be an objective to be approached on an all-or-nothing basis. Seen this way, it provides a target toward which any state or local home care agency can aspire.

3

Cost Analysis in Home Care

How to determine the costs associated with home care services accurately and comprehensively is of increasing concern to home care providers, government agencies, and third-party payers. Up to now, there has been a surprisingly wide degree of variation in defining which costs have been included in assessing home care programs, how these costs should be calculated, and what standardized quantity of service should be used to compare costs. This chapter focuses on these important issues for non-Medicare-certified home care agencies. It was prepared with the assistance of the National HomeCaring Council, where considerable research in the area of cost determinations has been carried out (Shinn, 1984).

DEFINING UNIT COSTS

An important beginning point in cost analysis is the definition of unit costs. A unit cost is the dollar cost of delivering one unit of service. Unit costs are typically computed by dividing the total cost associated with an activity by a measure of the services provided. This can be summarized by the equation

$$\frac{\text{Total Cost of Service}}{\text{Units of Service Provided}} = \text{Unit Cost}$$

Unit costs, defined in this way, provide a single, uniform measure with which to examine the relationship between the service delivered and the dollars spent on it.

A major problem in calculating unit costs for home care services stems from differences in the definition of what constitutes the service and which items of expense are included in it. This lack of standardization arises because the many public and private entities that provide home care have for the most part developed and operated independently. No overall governing body or standard-setting agency oversees their activities. Without at least some degree of standardization, however, many desirable applications using unit-cost analysis are not feasible. For example, in arriving at a competitive decision on a contract for services, differences in definitions of unit of service across bids may make comparative analysis difficult.

The following sections discuss some of the major variations that may be encountered in defining the components of home care service and the units that can be used to measure their provision.

SERVICE COMPONENTS

One important issue in cost analysis is the way in which agency administrative costs are handled. Agency administration includes all of the activities and resources required to support a provider agency and maintain it as a vehicle through which services are rendered. It includes the administrative functions of fundraising, office management, program planning, research, public relations, community involvement, evaluation and monitoring, personnel management, accounting, and bookkeeping. It also includes occupancy of an office site, maintenance, supplies, equipment, and other items related to maintaining a viable institution authorized to render a service and capable of being held accountable for funds and services.

Service administration, a second major component, is made

up of two subcomponents—case management and service management. Case management is focused on a specific case and includes intake, case supervision, and quality assurance. Service management refers to the overall administration of the service delivery function and includes scheduling, recruitment, training, and evaluation of worker performance.

Case management constitutes one of the areas in which there is the greatest variability and ambiguity in cost analysis, since agency practices and roles vary widely in this area. As discussed in Chapter 1, some public agencies contract out both the case management function and the direct-service delivery function to the provider agency, and some contract out only the service delivery function while retaining the case management responsibility themselves. Some even delegate these two functions to two separate sets of outside agencies, as in the case of Connecticut, discussed later in this chapter. Definitions of what is included in case management functions performed by vendor agencies and supervising agencies vary and sometimes involve ambiguity or overlap. An important task, therefore, for effective home care management is to define clearly the case management responsibilities of each participating agency and to measure accurately the costs of each function. Important for this purpose, and for assuring quality client service, is to define responsibilities for assisting clients with ancillary problems, ranging from managing their funds to arranging needed medical care and transportation, to dealing with housing problems, to making adjustments in the tasks provided by the home care worker. In analyzing the total costs of service, and in comparing different programs, such costs need to be accounted for whether incurred by the provider agency or the supervising agency.

The third component of home care service encompasses the activities of direct-service workers. All tasks performed for the client according to the plan of care—such as laundry, shopping, and participating in case conferences—should be included, as should travel costs, if workers are paid for travel to and from the client's home. So should other non-case-specific costs, if they have a valid connection to program expenditures.

Home care agencies vary as to which aspects of the three components of service they perform. Some agencies may perform all functions in each component, while other agencies may perform only some of the functions. Because this variation exists, it is very important to determine the scope of service of two agencies before comparing their unit costs. For example, one agency may perform the case management function of case assessment and may also develop the plan of care, while another agency may only do case intake. Another organization, such as an Area Agency on Aging, might handle all of the case management functions but rely on a provider agency to deliver the actual service. To avoid the "apples and oranges" comparison problem, it is essential to identify which functions are and are not included in an agency's service and cost data.

SERVICE UNITS

Several different types of units can be used to measure the volume of home care service, including time, people, and activities. What follows is an attempt to identify the principal variations in definitions of units of service and to point out their advantages and disadvantages.

Time

Time is a basic service dimension. It is the unit of service most commonly used by agencies to describe the level of service provided. Time can be defined as a service unit in terms of direct-service hours, all service hours, or service hours per case. Direct-service hours account only for the activities of the home aide. Service hours is a broader term and includes both the indirect activities of agency staff related to a case and the direct service of the home care worker.

At present, it appears that the direct-service hour is the most commonly used concept of the unit of service in home care. While this unit stands the greatest chance of being counted uniformly, it raises a number of definitional issues. For example, should travel time to and from the client's home be included? Should the time spent by an aide on case reporting be included? Should on-site supervision time of a case manager be included? The most common current practice is to count only that period of time that an aide spends in a client's home or in helping the client on such errands as laundry, shopping, or medical visits. Time spent on other services directly related to a specific client (such as case recording, travel, or case planning) is not included. This approach does not directly reflect costs of such activities as case management and supervision.

Although the cost per direct hour of service may be lower in one agency, its overall cost per case may be higher because of either higher overhead costs or less effective case management. Another agency with higher direct costs may be able to achieve lower total costs per hour or per case. Total cost per service hour and cost per case are definitions of unit costs that account for these related costs.

Number of People Served

A second major type of service unit is the number of people served. This indicator requires a count of either individuals, families, cases, or households. Comparability is only possible when all agencies count the same unit and if common rules are followed with respect to duplicated or unduplicated counts. For example, if a person is ill, receives service, recuperates, and several months later becomes ill and receives service again, is the person to be counted once or twice? Either approach may be acceptable, provided the approach used is clearly identified and recorded in the same way for all of the activities being examined.

Another problem that arises in counting people is that the raw numbers do not always reflect substantial differences in frequency and duration of services rendered. For example, in one case a client might receive only a single visit of two hours while in another case the client might receive three hours of service three times a week for 20 weeks. While both situations could be counted as either one case or one person being served, they are far from being equivalent in effort, time, or cost.

Kinds of Services Performed

A third aspect of defining the unit of service is the nature of activities performed by the home care worker. Home care is not a standardized, uniform activity performed in the same way for every client. Thus one cannot assume that one hour of service is comparable to another simply because each reflects 60 minutes of a worker's time. Besides the category of work performed, it should also be considered what the complexity and level of the activities are. Either of these two components of a service hour may require a worker to have special skills or experience; these requirements could in turn have an effect on cost and the duration of service to be rendered.

In terms of complexity, service plans can vary markedly as to the activities to be performed by the worker. In one case, the plan may call for only a few tasks, perhaps of a housekeeping nature. In another, many different tasks might need to be performed, covering such activity areas as housekeeping, home management, child care, and personal care. Complexity can also vary in terms of the provision of services to special types of clients such as the mentally ill, the severely handicapped, or the developmentally disabled. Working with such clients requires special approaches to performing basic tasks, which can increase the complexity of services required.

In terms of the level of service, several categories of activity can be defined that reflect a different degree of sophistication and require special training, knowledge, skills, and experience. A worker performing activities classifiable in one or more of these categories would be providing a different service that might require a pay differential, thus affecting cost.

The matter of difference in complexity and level of service is an important consideration which is at times overlooked in bidding and contracting for home care services. When the nature of the home care services desired is not written clearly into the request for proposals or the contract, or when an "hour of service at the least cost" is the only criterion for arriving at a decision, then agencies with specially skilled, experienced staff capable of serving clients with special needs are placed at a disadvantage. This dilemma can be eased if greater recognition is given to the variations that exist in defining units of service for different types of clients or different service plans.

CALCULATING AND USING UNIT-COST DATA

To calculate unit costs accurately, it is necessary to adopt both a standardized unit of service and a uniform method for determining total expenditures. Home care agencies, governments, and third-party payers should clearly define which service components are reflected in the cost data as well as which items of expense are included. Cost data should include both direct *and* overhead costs. Direct costs are those costs directly related to service delivery such as the home care aide and the case manager. Overhead costs (sometimes called indirect costs) are those expenses that cannot readily be allocated to specific clients or activities but are needed to support the agency's overall home care program. Examples of overhead costs are office management, accounting, and maintenance.

The method for handling contributed time, donated funds, and client fees also needs to be standardized. In bidding for a government contract, some agencies apply these revenues and/or contributions to reduce the unit cost to be charged. However, for purposes of comparing the true, unsubsidized cost per unit of service, no such deductions should be made.

Whatever the measure used as a yardstick, unit-cost data provide a useful assessment of the efficiency of a proposed program. They help answer the question, How well does a home care service provider utilize resources to provide a reasonable level of service? Unit-cost data can be used as a basis for billing, budgeting, contracting, administrative planning, policy making, comparing alternative services, and monitoring performance. This information can be extremely useful to both home care agencies and third-party payers responsible for financing and assuring cost-efficient service delivery.

For the home care agency, unit cost can become the basic billing unit per hour of service rendered. Where nondirect costs are reimbursed separately from direct costs, or the agency's fee is calculated after the service is delivered, total expenditures are likely to be fully recovered. However, if the unit cost is estimated prior to service delivery, as is usually the case in bidding and competitive contracting, then the degree of accuracy achieved in projecting the anticipated cost per hour of service becomes crucial. If the expense of providing an hour of service is either under- or overestimated in developing the prospective budget, revenue may not match actual expenses.

Unit costs can also be used as a basic budgeting tool in home care programs. Knowledge of the cost of delivering a unit of service during a previous budget period is an essential starting point in the process of arriving at a new budget, as it allows one to estimate the future per unit of service. Because they reflect both expenses and volume of service, unit-cost data can help managers make better informed projections.

Agencies can also use unit-cost data to improve internal management and planning capabilities by providing a clear definition of the costs of various agency activities and as a means of estimating the cost consequences of expanding or contracting a service area. Such information can also be used as a yardstick for assessing specific dimensions of agency performance as compared to those of other similar agencies.

Governments and other third-party payers can use unit-cost figures to compare costs among provider agencies that carry out comparable program activities. As the competition for home care resources increases, unit costs can be used as a tool to assist decision makers in choosing among prospective service providers.

Unit-cost figures can also enable governmental agencies to carry out performance-based monitoring and evaluation. Such information can be used to guide the day-to-day relationships between the agencies and the providers with whom they contract. It can also be used to identify contract agencies that require assistance in fiscal administration or program operations. By using a data base on unit costs, states or localities purchasing home care services can analyze factors associated with varying unit costs among providers. For example, cost per service hour can be analyzed in terms of the auspice, type, size, or certification status of a provider. Other factors whose cost implications can be analyzed include urban or rural location, sources of revenue, types of client served, skill level of aides used, and level of fringe benefits. Where an agency appears to display atypical cost patterns along a given dimension, assistance can be provided to help it overcome its problems and achieve results closer to the average cost for all providers.

COST COMPARISONS AND CLIENT CHARACTERISTICS

In comparing the costs of programs, differences in the programs need to be borne in mind. One dimension on which programs vary widely is the quantity of service provided to each client per unit time, that is, the number of hours of service per week or per month. These differences are often correlated with differences in the levels of impairment typical of the clients served by a given program. A program providing many hours of service per week may be serving a population of clients with very severe disabilities, requiring extensive assistance with such basic activities of daily living as ambulation, toileting, or feeding. The presence of incontinence, for example, can have a dramatic impact on the extent of home care needed.

The more impaired a client population is, the more likely it is that the clients served would actually have required and utilized institutional care such as a nursing home in the absence of the home care service. Similarly, where institutional care would otherwise have been required, the level and hence the cost of such care would be greater. A client who can feed herself, ambulate with mechanical aids, and get to the toilet on her own, but who needs help with bathing and dressing, might require a board-and-care or intermediate-care facility, while one who is incontinent and cannot ambulate without assistance would require a more expensive skilled nursing home if home care was not available. A client who needs only household tasks performed might well not actually utilize institutional care, even in the absence of home care, while a home care client whose impairment level is comparable to that of skilled nursing facility patients and who does not have family members available to provide help would almost certainly require some other form of care. Thus, comparisons of service allocations, and therefore of program costs on a per-case basis, require interpretation in the context of information on client characteristics to be most meaningful.

These types of data feed directly back to consideration of policy decisions relating to ceilings on the amount of hours to be authorized and procedures for authorization of the amount of service. Programs that have a relatively low ceiling on hours per week or month will have, almost by definition, low average hours per case and therefore low costs per case. Interpretation of these differences, however, requires knowledge of the profile of clients served. Such programs, for example, may not be able to provide adequate care for the severely impaired who require extensive assistance with personal care or constant attendance, and such clients may be considered unsuitable for home care. This may mean that the clients served by such a program typically may be considerably less impaired than those served by a program permitting more extensive service. One sort of policy decision facing home care policy makers is whether to provide service relatively thinly over a large number of clients or to provide more extensive care to a smaller number of severely impaired clients who most need care and who are most likely otherwise to require institutional care. Such decision making needs to be supported by adequate management information encompassing both fiscal and client-characteristics data.

The goal of integrated information management applies in this area as in others. Relatively few programs have yet been able systematically to integrate information on client characteristics, functional capabilities and impairments, and care needs with fiscal and other aspects of management information. The increasing availability of computers and utilization of computerized information systems in home care makes this type of integration an increasing possibility, however. Among the examples discussed in this book, the Alameda County approach represents perhaps the most significant model for such integration of client characteristics and needs data with other management information. In that model, data on the tasks with which the client needs assistance are used in a computer-based system to help determine service allocations, and the data become part of a data base that can be manipulated for analytic purposes, budget planning, and projections.

With such a computer-based system, for example, the financial impact of a policy decision to change service allocations to particular types of clients can be readily projected and fed back to the budgeting process. Thus, such systems can provide an ongoing way in which the impact of policies can be modeled and projected. The potential is created for a variety of analyses. Data become available on such issues as the cost per case for different types of cases. Data on the comparability of home care and institutional clients are particularly relevant. For example, by linking client impairment data with information on eligibility requirements of nursing home screening programs, one could compute the cost of home care for clients who are eligible for skilled nursing facility care and then compare that cost to skilled nursing facility costs. A similar analysis could be done for clients eligible for intermediate-care facilities. Such analyses (done at one point as a special study for New York City cases) could be produced on an ongoing basis, using current case load data.

CURRENT APPLICATIONS

A number of states and localities are using unit-cost data to strengthen fiscal management in their home care programs. For example, the Texas Department of Human Resources has developed a statewide uniform reimbursement rate for primary home care. Rates are determined on a statewide basis, using financial and statistical information from annual cost reports which must be submitted by each participating contractor. These are verified through on-site audits. The methodology for calculating unit costs presents reported expense data in a consistent manner, in order to determine allowed costs per hour. Adjustments are made in allowable costs to ensure that all costs used for rate setting are required for the primary home care service. Reimbursement rates are then prospectively determined for the coming year by projecting expenses from the past year. The reimbursement rate is based on the sum of projected expenses in three categories: field supervision, primary home care worker expense, and all other expenses. The allowable expense for each category is based on the 60th percentile of costs in that area across agencies in the previous year. This uniform unit rate is then used to reimburse all providers unless the contractor's customary charge is less than the state's reimbursement rate for the same service.

The Georgia Department of Medical Assistance makes payments to home care providers by using a prospective reimbursement system. Under this system, rates are initially determined based on historical cost information and a comparison of similar services provided by contractors. Thereafter, rates are adjusted to account for economic conditions and trends. Georgia's prospective system was developed to overcome some of the problems and inequities of the budgeted line-item reimbursement procedure. The system was designed to achieve more equitable rates among agencies, eliminate the year-end audit and cost settlement process, and permit greater control of government funds for home care.

In the State of Washington, a fixed unit rate is determined and used in all contracts for home care service. The contracts are performance-based in the sense that the provider is paid for the number of hours of service delivered rather than some proportion of budgeted operating expenses. A firm, fixed rate is set, largely based on cost data from the previous year, adjusted for economic trends.

The Pennsylvania Department on Aging has developed an accounting manual that provides the framework for a uniform cost-accounting system for all services administered by the state's Area Agencies on Aging. Such standardized accounting procedures facilitate planning, budgeting, and evaluation among cost centers and service activities at both the local and state levels.

In Iowa, the State Department of Health has required all home care agencies receiving departmental funds to calculate and report unit costs in a uniform manner. The uniform format enables the department to compare specific cost components such as fringe benefits, administration, and direct services on an interagency basis. Costs are analyzed by type of agency, auspice, size, and a number of other factors. Using this analysis, statewide norms for various cost components are established. These guidelines have been used to identify agencies whose cost patterns differ substantially from the norm. Technical assistance has been offered to these more costly agencies, to help them bring their costs in line with the norm.

The key to developing a useful system of unit-cost measurement is uniformity in defining the central issues. All participants must agree on what constitutes the service rendered, what is counted in an hour of service, and what expenses are used to establish cost. Once these issues are resolved and cost data become standardized, the use of unit costs in analyzing home care programs can have a significant impact on the provision of service and on the relationship between funding sources and providers.

4

Staffing and Personnel Practices

The public administrator who funds home care services, the worker who provides the service, and the client who receives the service can have differing views on staffing and personnel practices. The one-to-one nature of home care service delivery makes it a very labor-intensive service. Thus, costs for direct-service personnel are particularly dominant in total home care costs. Decisions on staffing and personnel issues affect the current and future supply of able and willing workers.

The wages and benefits of home care workers and their training, staff development, and scheduling are interrelated with the fiscal management issues discussed in Chapter 2. Decisions on the allocation of hours and services, rate setting, and/or utilization patterns are often driven by costs related to compensation and training, by the availability or supply of workers, and by the openness of agencies and workers to flexible scheduling. Successful integration of funding streams may depend upon the generic training of home care workers capable of performing both homemaker and home health aide tasks. On the other hand, the use of generically trained workers with no extra pay for specialization may delay the development of a career ladder within home care. New computer technologies can provide the management information necessary to facilitating efficient scheduling as well as faster submission of claims and prompt timesheet processing, which assures timely payment of workers.

Because the home care field has grown so fast and programs vary so greatly across states, localities, and agencies, few national empirical data exist on personnel issues. This chapter draws upon data obtained through the Home Care Fiscal Management Project and upon what little national research exists.

WAGES AND BENEFITS

The compensation paid to home care workers constitutes the major cost of home care. Wages, downtime, overtime and benefits are in turn the principal determinants of total worker compensation. Ninety percent of the rate paid to New York City home attendant vendors goes to the home attendants as wages and fringes, both for time in the client's home and for vacation, sick pay, training, and other non-client-care time. Policies that determine the amount of non-client-care time are major factors in determining cost; for example, Iowa's Department of Health reported to the Home Care Fiscal Management Project that their financial analyses indicate that the largest source of variance in hourly costs among agencies was due to the amount of non-client-care time for which workers were paid.

In many areas of the country, home care workers are hourly workers paid at, or just above, the minimum wage. They can be paid even less under certain circumstances. In Oklahoma workers receive a flat daily rate to accomplish assigned tasks, which may work out to less than minimum wage. An Alameda County In-Home Supportive Services (IHSS) worker may negotiate with clients for a flat monthly rate, with room and board, for 24-hour coverage, which can also work out to be less than minimum wage. In a few metropolitan areas, such as New York City or San Francisco, unions have gained the right to bargain in home care agencies to improve pay and benefits for home care workers. The unions that represent home care workers in New York City negotiated a new contract for 1986 for a base pay of $4.15 an hour, with regular increments based on length of service. In Connecticut virtually all home care services are obtained through the private sector, whether proprietary or nonprofit, and wages are largely determined by the market.

The issue of overtime is a growing problem for many states because the needs of the client may not fit neatly into a 40-hour week. Decisions concerning overtime, particularly for companion-type care, have not been consistent among federal regional offices. New York State law allows certain nonprofit agencies to be exempt from overtime requirements. New York City home attendants who are present in the client's home for 24 hours are paid on the basis of 12 hours a day, unless care must be provided throughout the night, in which case two shifts of workers are provided. The state and city are trying to limit these dual-shift cases, particularly for new cases being released from hospitals. This has caused younger, severely physically disabled persons to be fearful they may be forced to return to chronic-care hospitals or will not be able to be discharged to independent living. Texas contractors, working under unit rates, avoid paying any overtime by hiring multiple providers. Alameda County workers are not authorized to be paid to work over 40 hours a week. This serves to avoid overtime payment, although, as mentioned earlier, workers may negotiate for live-in care.

Benefits for home care workers may include Social Security (FICA); Worker's Compensation; Unemployment Insurance; pensions; health coverage; travel and uniform reimbursement; and paid holidays, sick leave, and annual leave. Whether any or all of these benefits are paid, and by whom, depends on the workers' employment status, individual state and local policies, and the presence or absence of unions. Texas contractors will even schedule workers in such a way as to keep their weekly hours low enough to avoid having to pay some mandated benefits.

It is unusual for home care workers to be paid for holidays and annual and sick leaves, in full or prorated. In New York City, part-time home attendants employed by vendor agencies receive prorated sick and annual leave but no holidays; full-time workers receive all three, as well as health insurance. Retirement benefits are rarer still.

Other employee benefits may include reimbursement of travel between assignments as well as the provision of uniforms. It is usual, but not universal, for agencies to pay for travel between assignments, which can be a considerable expense in sparsely populated areas or where public transportation is costly or limited. The National HomeCaring Council recommends that agencies that require uniforms should provide them if the worker is only paid minimum wage.

Employers are required to pay Federal Insurance Contributions Act (FICA) taxes for any worker who earns over $50 a quarter. At issue is who pays FICA taxes, as well as Worker's Compensation and Unemployment Insurance, if the worker is an "independent provider" and not on the payroll of a public or private agency. If the client is considered the employer, must the client withhold the employee share and provide the employer portion, while typically being on some kind of public assistance herself or himself? And if the worker is injured on the job, does the client's liability insurance (if any) cover the injury, or is it covered by Worker's Compensation? These issues are discussed further in the next chapter.

Home care workers who are Civil Service workers and receive regular increments and some or all of the benefits discussed previously are usually considered by public administrators to be more expensive than independent providers or workers in contract agencies. This is one of the reasons states such as Iowa have shifted to contracting in recent years.

The lack of a career ladder within home care service has been a problem. In many areas of the country the custom has been to pay the same rate for workers regardless of whether clients needed only housekeeping and meal preparation or needed more complicated personal care tasks requiring specialized skills. The rationale was that the same worker would be able to continue to care for clients whose needs changed, thereby sparing the clients the trauma of losing familiar workers. In recent years public administrators have been unwilling to provide highly trained workers to do only housekeeping services at the same rate as workers performing more complex services. The response has been either to set up separate, less costly housekeeping or chore services, as has been done in Washington State, or to set up special high-paid cadres of workers.

This has had the effect of creating a career ladder of sorts. In Texas more skilled workers do not require the same high level of on-site orientation and are able to serve the more difficult clients. They can be trusted to provide care before a supervisor is able to go into the home to assess the situation and assign an aide. These more highly skilled workers may be able to command higher pay. However, rather than directing a career ladder approach, the Texas Department of Human Resources outlines the need for such workers in their request for contractors' proposals and invites potential contractors to use their creativity and propose solutions. New York City's Human Resources Administration is designing a special program for home care for adult protective services that calls for higher pay as well as increased training and supervision for the workers.

These compensation issues have been and will continue to be of particular interest to women, because home care is a low-paying field dominated by women. A National Research Council study (1985), funded by the Carnegie Corporation and the U.S. Departments of Education and of Labor, reported that the representation of women as nursing aides, a low-paying job similar to that of home care workers, was 87.0% in 1970 and 87.8% in 1980.

STAFF DEVELOPMENT AND TRAINING

Public administrators must decide if they will require and fund training of home care workers, supervisors, and/or administrators. If they do, they must decide who should provide the training and what should be its content. Beyond the cost of the training itself, there are other fiscal implications. Do training and staff development contribute to aides', supervisors', and administrators' more efficient and effective functioning? Are regrettable incidents of negligence, which can be costly, due to inadequate training?

Public administrators and home care agency directors differ on whether formal aide training is necessary or even desired. Because of the frailty of home care clients, some administrators are becoming more concerned over the skill level of home care workers who are either employed by contract agencies or who are individual providers. For home care programs they fund, Iowa's Department of Health, North Carolina's Division of Social Services, the State of Rhode Island, and South Carolina's Commission on Aging and Department of Social Services require the use of the National HomeCaring Council's Model Curriculum (National HomeCaring Council, 1980) or a program equivalent in content and depth. New York State and Arkansas require training for aides modeled after the National HomeCaring Council's standards for home care agency accreditation: 60 hours of generic training within the first six months, 16 hours of which should be completed before going into a client's home, and 40 hours of which should be completed before providing any personal care. The standards also call for a minimum of 8 hours of inservice training a year. The National HomeCaring Council has published a training manual for home care workers who work with the developmentally disabled. It has also produced three other publications geared to the special training needs of workers—one on care for cancer patients, one for high-tech home care, and one for high-risk infants.

Both New York City and Washington, D.C., have observed that the skill level of their new workers is lower than before. Because of this, the New York City Medical Assistance Program now requires all new home attendants to complete two days of preservice training in body mechanics and personal care. These are two of five training modules approved by the New York State Department of Social Services. Home attendants are tested on all five modules and certified if they pass. If they fail one or more of the three other modules, the workers are allowed to begin work, with 90 days to pass the failed module(s). If they fail just one of the two preservice modules they may repeat the training and be reimbursed for car fare. If they pass both modules the first time, they can be reimbursed for their 2 days in training. If they fail both preservice modules, they are dropped. The city contracts with several agencies to provide this training, while home care agencies are responsible for providing half-day inservice training twice a year.

Home care agencies are beginning to worry about being sued because of insufficient aide training (Nassif, 1985). Liability suits in home care are beginning to appear in lower courts, naming individual providers, agencies, counties, cities, and/or states for negligence. Liability is created by the "doctrine of ostensible agency," that is, the appearance that a worker is controlled and supervised by an agency. This can include agency volunteers. In Wisconsin's consumer-directed county services programs, the worker is considered the client's employee; nevertheless, counties have been sued for liability in injury cases (Silverberg, 1984). In this environment all agency workers—aides, supervisors, and administrators—must learn to document fully every incident, to be prepared in the event of lawsuits. With the advent of DRG's and sicker clients requiring more high-tech care, charges of negligence will increase. This has implications for the level of training home care workers will require. Alameda County already reports serving sicker clients as a result of DRG's in California, but it still requires no training for its self-employed workers.

A related training and liability issue concerns state nurse practice acts. These acts prohibit home care workers who are employed in an agency and supervised by nurses from performing certain "health-related tasks," even if they have been trained to perform them. If workers are considered employees of the client, they can be trained and supervised by nurses to give diabetes shots or provide such other health-related tasks as catheter or tracheostomy tube care. At issue is the nurse's liability if she actually supervises an employee in the performance of these tasks. Home care agencies are not able to obtain liability insurance if their paraprofessionals are performing any of these health-related tasks. Through exemptions to nurse practice acts, aides in mental health institutions are often allowed to administer medications.

Public administrators complain that rapid turnover of home care workers means a loss of their training investment. For this reason, some administrators are unwilling to pay for training. They also contend that mature women who have raised their own families need little or no training or that the training that nurse's aides receive in hospitals or nursing homes is sufficient for them as home care workers. In either instance, they argue, whatever else workers need to know can be taught by nurses or social workers on the job. An opposing view is that former nurse's aides need additional formal training in home care techniques because their hospital or nursing home training has prepared them to work only under direct, physically present, professional supervision. Although Texas does not require any specific training curriculum for home care workers, workers there must demonstrate competence in personal care before being allowed to provide it. If necessary, supervisors then give on-the-job training to correct any deficiencies.

Administrators in home care and in long-term care do not all agree on the definition of case management. Some experts in the field maintain that supervision of the worker is one of the case-specific functions of case management, in addition to such customary functions as eligibility determination, assessment, and care planning. However, the common pattern of supervision in publicly financed home care is for the public agency to retain what it considers to be its case management responsibilities for the client, with either the home care agency or the client supervising the work of the home care provider.

The National HomeCaring Council and the Brookdale Center on Aging at Hunter College (both in New York City) each have published curricula on aide supervision. Brookdale's curriculum contains modules on helping aide supervisors to recognize special behavior problems, especially of the elderly, and to understand cultural needs and differences. Texas takes the position that it is more cost effective for all training efforts to be directed to agency supervisors rather than to home care workers. Texas requires 14 hours of training for supervisors in basic supervision, interpersonal skills, and client characteristics and needs, with 6 hours of ongoing training each quarter, to include how supervisors can improve workers' skills. The workers are supervised on site every other month and are trained by supervisors to correct any deficiencies. When Texas contracted with vendor agencies in its Medicaid personal care program, some public agency case managers were reluctant to turn over completely the supervision of the aides to the contract agencies. Since the state was purchasing aide supervision as part of its contracts, this presented a cost issue of case manager time lost to the state.

Both Connecticut Community Care, Inc. (CCCI) and the New School for Social Research in New York have recognized the need for formal training for case managers. CCCI's training, an interdisciplinary approach to case management for nurses and social workers, includes leveraging services and funding sources, developing service contracts and information support systems, and the use of an assessment instrument. The New School developed a certificate program in case management for the elderly in its School of Management and Urban Professions. Such training could be useful for case managers of home care clients in the public sector, as well as for case managers in home care contract agencies where functions other than aide supervision are purchased.

In the past, home care administrators were apt to come from the "helping professions" of nursing or social work and sometimes lacked the requisite management skills. In the late 1970s the Administration on Aging funded the National HomeCaring Council to develop a cadre of management experts as trainers and consultants for agency administrators and to conduct management institutes to improve agency efficiency and effectiveness. Modules on personnel and staff development, wage and salary administration, budgeting, legal issues, data collection and evaluation procedures, use of computers, marketing, and organizational structure and change were presented throughout the country.

SCHEDULING

The scheduling of home care workers is closely related to the allocation of hours. Many agencies require a minimum of four hours for a visit, thereby reducing costly down time and guaranteeing a certain number of hours of work for the worker. However, the periods of time home care is needed by a client do not always match agency or worker needs. Clients often need help in evenings, early mornings, and weekends, for short periods of time (Kane, 1985). Kane called on agencies to be willing to create flexible schedules and questioned whether government and taxpayers should pay for costly four-hour minimums. New York City is considering requiring flexible scheduling capacity for some adults in need of protection, to meet their particular needs at certain times of the day. Proprietary agencies are even beginning to advertise that they will provide care in less than four-hour blocks of time.

In areas where clients live close together, agencies are experimenting with clustering home care workers. Several aides can be assigned to a housing project and can provide care to several clients during the day. New York's Monroe County Social Services Agency has demonstrated the cost effectiveness of such an approach. Home attendants are assigned in clusters to a United Cerebral Palsy apartment house in New York City, through a vendor agency contract.

Good computerized management information systems can provide necessary and timely data on client, service, and personnel statistics, in order to assist schedulers in assigning workers more efficiently, matching client needs, worker skills, and geographic locations. Management information systems are used to support scheduling in this fashion in Wake County, North Carolina.

Electronic call buttons and other such emergency response systems as supplements to home care can be cost-effective devices that help relieve the anxiety of clients living alone, as well as the fears of their families. Texas uses these devices widely, and

New York City is experimenting with their use in selected cases, as a solution to the need for 24-hour availability. False alarms, sometimes caused because of memory loss, can limit their usefulness to only those clients who can remember to reset the devices and to press them in times of emergency. A nonprofit program, Life Safety Systems, provides direct, around-the-clock protection in case of fire and medical emergency for homebound persons, particularly the elderly. Developed by the International Association of Fire Fighters in partnership with the Muscular Dystrophy Association, the system is tied into municipal fire departments that serve as communications centers, eliminating the need for often costly third-party monitoring. Life Safety Systems is headquartered in Washington, D.C. Participating communities presently include Pittsburgh, Pennsylvania; Anaheim, California; San Antonio, Texas; Topeka, Kansas; Montgomery County, Maryland; and Phoenix, Arizona.

SUPPLY OF WORKERS

Conversations with public administrators indicate that the supply of home care workers in their areas relates to the local economy and employment opportunities for lower-income workers. For the future, the supply depends on the rate of growth of the demand for home care, as well as on the economy. Unknown is whether the changing role of women in the workplace will bring about a mismatch between available, willing, and capable workers and the number of home care jobs available.

Those areas of the country that are experiencing shortages of workers report a strengthening of their local economy. As the "baby boom" shrinks, their service industries are turning to older workers, particularly in suburban areas. Home care agencies may have to improve their wages and benefits to compete and retain experienced workers. With low unemployment rates in their areas, the Connecticut Department on Aging and the Massachusetts Executive Office of Elder Affairs report pronounced shortages. Connecticut's Department of Education has established an ad hoc task force of educators, health providers, and state agency personnel to identify the needs of health-related personnel for the future and to establish education programs to meet the need.

Massachusetts cites competition in the state outside Boston, from both the high-tech industries and such service employers as McDonald's. State officials reported that nursing homes are experiencing similar problems. To meet this problem they are looking to paying higher wages and improved benefits and to requiring contract home care agencies to provide health insurance coverage. For the first time Massachusetts has allowed Home Care Corporations to hire their own homemakers as staff to serve in emergencies and fill gaps, thereby guaranteeing them employment. These homemakers are used where there are worker shortages and also to provide more rapid service response to elders discharged from hospitals. This is particularly important because of the increase in the intensity of needs brought on by the DRG reimbursement system. The on-staff worker can deliver service the day the elder returns home, rather than after the normal delay in contacting agencies, locating workers, and initiating services.

New York City finds that availability and retention of capable aides are problems in some areas of the city and fears they may become more problematical in the future, depending upon the economy. New York vendor agencies also report difficulties finding and retaining nurses as supervisors because of competition from higher paying certified home health agencies, proprietary home care agencies, hospitals, and nursing homes.

As it was experiencing an economic recession in 1986, Texas had no difficulties finding workers. Supervisors were able to tap informal neighborhood networks for both skilled workers for difficult cases and less skilled workers. Alameda County experiences seasonal problems, competing with options offered in agriculture in the summer months, and with Christmas work in the late fall and early winter. Maine reports problems during blueberry picking and packing season. Resort areas in New York State lure home care workers to higher paying jobs during the summer.

In the future the supply of home care workers may be met partially through state requirements for welfare recipients to work. Through a federal grant, New Jersey's Department of Human Services demonstrated that training and placing AFDC mothers as homemakers was effective as long as the pay was sufficient and work was guaranteed, with regular hours. In many areas of the country in the 1970s, Comprehensive Employment and Training Act (CETA) programs served as sources of home care workers. With the expansion of home care, some workers found jobs when CETA was phased out.

Nursing homes and hospitals have also been sources of workers because home care agencies can offer flexible and part-time work to nurse's aides who may need to work around their children's schedule or who just want to supplement their incomes. However, institutions also hire workers away from home care agencies because they can guarantee a full work week and regular hours. This is important for those who must work full time as the sole support of their families.

As discussed earlier, home care workers are usually mature women. In large urban areas and certain other areas of the country, they are apt to be minority women who are supporting families. Home care programs can provide many jobs and be important to the economy of the area, as are other health-related entry-level jobs. Furthermore, since women have dominated the nursing and social work fields, home care supervisors are also usually women. However, with improved job opportunities for some women, questions about the future supply of workers suitable for home care jobs have been raised. This is already being seen in teaching and in child care jobs. In some urban areas there has been no shortage of female minority home care workers because of poor economic conditions and high immigration from Third World countries. The imposition of penalties on employers for hiring undocumented aliens under legislation effective in 1987 may lead to some shortages of home care workers in both urban and rural areas. Nonetheless, the apparent lack of concern among most public administrators and planners for long-term care reflects their belief that there will be an inexhaustible pool of low-income women able and willing to fill these jobs. It is doubtful that men would be considered suitable as home care workers of the majority of clients, who are elderly women living alone.

There is no doubt that the demand for home care will grow, but projections of the rate of growth differ. Seldom has the issue of the adequacy of the future supply of workers to meet this growth been analyzed in detail. The U.S. Department of Labor (USDOL) examined the issue and projected the number of home care workers that would be needed by 1990, using several alternative sets of assumptions about the demand for home care (Terlizzi, 1977). These projections assumed the continuation of a high employee turnover rate, as is typical of this and other occupations that do not require highly developed skills or specific formal education. Terlizzi's analysis raises questions as to whether enough workers will be available to meet the demand for home care, even under the most conservative projection of demand. Her proposed solution was to make the job more secure, with higher wages, benefits, and prestige and more opportunities for advancement and peer support. These solutions all have cost implications for home care. Terlizzi also projected that employment opportunities for nurses and social workers would grow faster than traditional employment opportunities through 1990.

Long-term care settings may be at an increasing recruiting disadvantage. To overcome an acute shortage of nurses for hospitals in the mid 1970s, salaries for hospital nurses were raised to an average of $25,000 to $35,000 per year by 1985–1986. Nurses' salaries tend to be lower in long-term care than in hospitals; this has implications for the numbers of nurses who will be willing to work as case managers or supervisors in home care. Enrollment in schools of nursing is also declining throughout the country (Oriol, 1985).

Questioning USDOL's assumptions, Weissert (1985b) states that, even if a broader definition of dependency than being eligible for nursing home placement were used, it would not produce the demand for home care that many anticipate. Weissert concludes that projections to the year 2000 of overall prevalence of functional dependency will "remain smaller than popularly believed" and that the demand for home care services and workers in many areas of the country will not grow as much as projected. He claims that only larger cities now can produce sufficient numbers of dependent elderly eligible for nursing homes to support long-term community care demonstrations.

Home care is a highly personal, labor-intensive service whose quality ultimately depends on the skill and attitudes of the individual worker. It is precisely the individual, personal aspect of home care that brings with it both the potential for a far more satisfying experience than institutional care and the risk of unsupervised inadequacies or even abuses. The more routinized quality of life and care in institutionalized settings affords closer employee supervision but often removes the sense from patients that the locus of control vests with them, and can be dissatisfying for health care workers as well. The situation places more responsibility on the worker, since supervision is inherently more remote in the home care situation. Administrators must trade off the value of more extensive training and supervision against its costs and against the risk that making home care more expensive could ultimately make it less feasible as an alternative to institutional care. Thus, personnel practices require careful attention and ongoing monitoring as to their effects.

5

Employer–Employee Relationships in Independent Provider Programs

In many home care programs, the worker providing services is considered an "independent provider," not an employee of a public or private home care agency. In such programs, the relationships among workers, clients, and the agencies providing the funds are legally ambiguous. Who is the employer when the worker is considered an individual provider? Is the worker the employee of the client? Or is the worker an independent contractor and therefore self-employed? And what is the employment status of family members paid to care for their relatives?

BACKGROUND: RECENT STUDIES

There have been a few recent studies that have looked at the issues surrounding independent provider programs, including those that employ family members. This chapter discusses the employee-employer issues raised in these studies and draws on state and local experiences both from these studies and from research undertaken in the Home Care Fiscal Management Project.

A grant to the National HomeCaring Council underwrote research on individual providers (Layzer, 1981). This research outlined the common-law tests of employment and analyzed the strengths and weaknesses of individual provider programs. Common law sets out a number of tests to determine the employment relationship; however, states have varied in their interpretations of these tests. The tests include (1) who controls the number of hours of care and how and when care is provided; (2) who has the right to hire and fire, set the salary, and pay the worker; (3) who pays for the supplies, tools, or facilities; (4) whether there is permanency; (5) whether or not the work is part of the employer's regular business; and, finally, (6) whether or not there is belief by either party that an employer-employee relationship has been created. If the client is the employer, it is hard to ensure FICA coverage for the employee. To overcome this, the Social Security Administration and the Internal Revenue Service have been encouraging states to act as "agents" for the client/employer (sec. 3504 IRS Code and Revenue Procedure 80-4). However, some states are unwilling to do so, to avoid the appearance of assuming "employer-like" responsibilities and therefore being held liable both for other benefits and for the actions of the workers. Payment mechanisms also vary by program and can include two-party checks that must be signed by both the client and workers; direct checks to the workers; and checks to clients, who then pay their workers. The mechanism selected also has implications for employer-like behavior.

The strengths and weaknesses of individual provider programs vary from the perspective of the client, provider, and taxpayer (Layzer, 1981). From the clients' perspective, the program provides them with independence and self-worth because they select and direct their workers. This is particularly important for younger, physically disabled clients who are capable of directing and training workers to meet their special needs. Where there is a dearth of agencies, as in sparsely populated rural areas, independent provider arrangements may be the only way that clients can get home care on weekends, in crisis situations, or at all. However, workers can be unreliable. Under such arrangements, it is often difficult for clients to select and screen workers and there is no agency to send in replacements in case of workers' illness or their quitting suddenly. There have been allegations of abuse and neglect in these programs because of reduced monitoring and supervision. The late Dr. Ellen Winston testified before both the Senate and House in 1975 that home care workers should not work as self-employed practitioners because of their level of training (Layzer, 1981).

From the workers' perspective, independent provider programs can reinforce the informal support system by paying family members who would otherwise have to work outside the home. Workers believe they can be paid more because no funds are going into administration; but workers may be provided with poor compensation, sometimes less than minimum wage, and few or no benefits. This has been characterized as reflecting sexism and racism in such programs, since most of the workers are women and often minority women.

There is no consensus on the economy of individual provider programs, whose true costs are often not recognized. Some believe the programs are cost-effective approaches because of savings on fringe benefits and administrative expenses. Others see them as more costly approaches that drive up case costs because of overutilization. Particularly if family members are used as providers, it is argued, overutilization may create more dependence because often there is little monitoring, training, and supervision. Since family members may view the reimbursement as an income supplement, they often resist reducing hours.

Employer-employee issues were raised in a study for the Health Care Financing Administration that examined the provision of financial incentives for family care allowed under the Social Services Block Grant programs, under Medicaid Section 2176 waivers, or through tax incentives (Burwell, 1986). These programs usually involve paying low-income family caregivers. Support for paying family members was reported to be growing among public administrators. The study also cited increased flexibility in scheduling, less turnover of workers, and perceived better quality of care. However, savings may have been realized because states have been lax in adherence to federal and state laws related to wages and benefits for family members. Of particular interest to the fiscal managers of home care is whether there is a substitution effect if family members are paid, that is, is the public agency paying for services that would have been provided by family members in any event? Allowing family members to receive reimbursement does not appear to increase net short-term substitution and may increase long-term incentives for family members to stay involved (Urban Systems Research and Engineering, 1982). However, Burwell's (1986) study concluded that the states that have substitution problems lack policy guidelines; have no limits on how much is paid, who can be paid, and for what; and have no requirements for prior approval. Unless there is adequate monitoring, he concluded, there is potential for abuse and neglect by family members.

Federal and state tax incentive programs are being considered as partial subsidies for leveraging privately financed services by family members. Such tax incentives are believed to be more appropriate in moderate-income families. Again, there is considerable concern over the great potential public cost unless targeting can be improved based on diagnosis and/or disability, income, and living arrangements. Some tax advantage for caretaking for dependent elderly already exists in the federal income tax.

STATE AND LOCAL EXPERIENCES

At one time or another, each of the five consortium sites discussed in this book has used independent providers. By the early 1980s, Texas, New York City, and Washington State had transferred all or a portion of their individual provider programs to contract programs involving provider agencies. Their interesting approaches to rate setting and contracting practices contributed to their selection as examples of innovative fiscal management practices. Their reasons for contracting were similar: (1) concern over federal and state interpretations of who was the actual employer for purposes of FICA, Worker's Compensation, Unemployment Insurance, income tax, and other related issues; (2) concern over the lack of supervision and its effect on the quality of service for the client and the lack of fiscal control for the public agency; and (3) concern over the burden placed on the client to find suitable caregivers and do the paperwork if the client were considered the employer. New York City had an additional reason: Their program had grown so rapidly that its administrative procedures had not kept pace with the program and home attendants were not being paid in a timely manner. This caused problems both for the attendants and the clients.

While the State of Washington's Chore Services program was changed over to a contract program, that state's Personal Care program has continued to use individual providers. The state is suffering from high unemployment; nonetheless, administrators report clients find it difficult to find suitable workers because of low pay and the lack of benefits. Furthermore, nurses are skeptical of the quality of care, which they now see as particularly critical since the DRG system is leading to release of some patients earlier and sicker. The state has found it difficult to control hours, a situation that is typical of independent contractor programs. One hundred percent of authorized hours are claimed, in comparison with a more common 90% of authorized hours actually delivered in contract programs in Washington State and elsewhere.

A difficult problem arose in the changeover to a contracted program in New York City. Some independent providers who had been performing certain health-related tasks (e.g., giving insulin shots) were not allowed to perform them as agency employees, because of state nurse practice acts. Although the city set up a third-party agency for the younger severely physically disabled, to provide back-up workers and handle payments and benefits, the health-related task problem remains. This issue has been difficult for advocates for the physically disabled to accept. Weisman (1985) asserted that some disabled individuals might have to be institutionalized at considerably greater cost to Medicaid if their attendants were no longer able to perform such tasks.

In the mid-1980s Connecticut vendorized its independent provider companion program. The transition was relatively simple because of the existence of a case management system. The issues were primarily focused on problems due to labor law; therefore, the contract agency was needed only for payrolling purposes. California still permits counties the option of service delivery through self-employed providers or by contracting with voluntary or proprietary agencies. Some counties permit all three. A California study (Wood & Rosen, 1980) identified many of the same problems in individual provider programs experienced in New York City and Texas and uncovered reports of abuse and exploitation in several areas of California. To overcome the problem of payroll systems that broke down frequently, California contracted out the payroll system and took over the statewide payment of workers, including FICA, Worker's Compensation, and Unemployment Insurance. They declared the state and recipient co-employers. Because the program does not pay benefits for spouses or parents, benefits for the independent providers average only 9 percent of direct wages, as contrasted with 12 to 22 percent for agency employees. Unemployment Insurance is paid if the worker is paid $72.01 a week for 18 weeks, but 68 percent of workers earn less than this.

Other states or localities have also shifted from independent providers to contracting for services. For example, Arkansas changed over because of lawsuits on Worker's Compensation. A multicounty area in western Kentucky moved to a contract program in the late 1970s because of a lawsuit on Unemployment Insurance at the same time that state funding for the program was reduced. Western Kentucky found in the course of vendorizing that, although funding was decreased and administrative expenses increased, training for case managers, an improved assessment and reassessment process, and increased levels of worker supervision resulted in fewer hours per client and allowed them to serve the same number of clients for less money.

The Personal Care program operated by Oklahoma's Department of Human Resources was still an independent provider program in the mid-1980s, apparently the oldest one in the country funded by Medicaid. Oklahoma classified individual providers as self-employed, so they did not have to be paid minimum wage. In April of 1983 staff reported a daily stipend of $13 a day, plus $0.97 for FICA, with the state acting as agent for the client just as California does. Providers agreed to work at least 3 hours a day but to work as many hours a day as are required to complete the care plan. They received 20 hours of training from registered nurses who supervised 100 to 105 clients each. Regulations called for a supervision visit every 60 days.

As of 1983 Missouri still allowed clients to choose providers either from independent providers or from public or private agencies in the state's Social Service Block Grant (SSBG) program. In the case of independent providers, payment was negotiated by the client and the worker, within a maximum of $295 a month, plus FICA. Two-party checks were mailed to the client, who payed the provider. Wisconsin has taken another approach in that state's county-administered Title XX Supportive Home

Care Program. Three-way service agreements among the county, client, and provider set out activities, schedules, billing procedures, and rates, the latter being negotiated between the provider and the county. Minimum payments in 1984 ranged widely among counties, from $50 a quarter to $640 a month. Where Unemployment Insurance coverage has been contested, the court has ruled that the county was the employer under the common-law test of employment. The basis for each of the rulings has been that the county had the right to control the work performed, even though the client might have had *de facto* control (Silverberg, 1984).

Employment policies with regard to family members as caregivers differ among states and even among counties within states (Burwell, 1986). The policies are a crazy-quilt of restricted and permitted arrangements. Some exclude family members who live with the client (to avoid substitution for already existing care), while others are just the opposite, excluding those family members who do *not* live with the client. Some policies restrict the amount of money that can be paid family members and/or require prior approval. Policies may stipulate which tasks can be reimbursed; those allowed are usually personal care tasks, that is, activities of daily living but not shopping and other instrumental activities of daily living.

The following state examples further illustrate the variety of approaches to the payment of family members as of 1985. Michigan, Maryland, and Kansas excluded spouses entirely. Virginia's Adult Services Program would pay family members for SSBG chore services at $3.35 an hour, provided they did not live with the client. On the other hand, Florida, Connecticut, North Dakota, and Maryland would only pay family members if they did live with the client. Florida's Home Care for the Elderly Program, funded by state dollars under Aging and Adult Services, allowed payment only for relatives who live with the client. In Connecticut close relatives were not reimbursed unless it could be documented that there was no other appropriate provider and the relative had been required to relinquish gainful employment. North Dakota's state-funded Family Home Care Program would pay up to $250 a month for moderate care and $375 for maximum care to relatives, provided the relative and client lived together. Kansas's Section 2176 program did not pay spouses except under special circumstances and required at least minimum wage. In Wisconsin, counties could exclude family members altogether or restrict their use to those who were employable. If prior approval was received, both Minnesota's Section 2176 program and Maine's Elderly Home Bound Care Program would allow payment of family members. Maine required special monitoring in such cases. Minnesota stipulated that payment of relatives be a last resort and that financial hardship be demonstrated. Live-in relatives could only be paid for a maximum of 40 hours a week in Oregon's Section 2176 waiver program.

Especially interesting are the developments that took place when Michigan shifted 75% of its Chore Services program in 1980 from Title XX funding to Medicaid Personal Care funding, as an optional service. Michigan defined family members as only those who are spouses and parents of minor children, which has allowed them to pay other relatives without a waiver. Texas has used the same definition of family as Michigan for its Personal Care program, based on state law defining responsibility for support. This definition for their Personal Care program has survived a Health Care Financing Administration (HCFA) challenge to the use of family members other than spouses and parents of minor children. Such extensive use of relatives is unusual under Title XIX; however, it is expected that more states may adopt this provision if it is not disallowed by HCFA.

Four states had adopted state tax incentive plans. Idaho, Oregon, Iowa, and Arizona were testing state tax incentives for family members to provide care. Oregon instituted a nonrefundable tax credit of 8% of eligible expenses, to a maximum of $250, with an income limit; Idaho allowed either a $1,000 deduction or a refundable tax credit of $100. Iowa permitted up to $5,000 in deductions from gross income, and Arizona allowed unlimited medical deductions and an additional $600 if deductions exceeded $800.

CONCLUSION

The use of independent provider arrangements to reimburse some family members of the care of others raises important, complex political and social issues concerning the interface of government and private roles in the care of the elderly. Do such arrangements constitute an unwarranted involvement of government in paying for family members to carry out their preexisting family responsibilities? Or do they represent a highly desirable synergism between the formal and informal caretaking systems, involving a cost-effective use of the latter to help the former attain its objectives? American values are not clear on these matters. While there appears to have been an attitudinal shift over the last three decades away from expectations of responsibilities of adult children for financial assistance of noncoresident parents (cf. Crystal, 1984), expectations concerning personal care responsibilities are not well defined. Payment for family care through independent-provider home care programs represents a rather little-known and little-studied, yet quite extensive, experiment in public subsidy for caregiving by family members. If extended to even a significant percentage of the large numbers who potentially could need and claim such assistance, these arrangements could indeed be far-reaching elements of social policy. Much more research on reimbursed family care arrangements is needed.

Independent provider arrangements represent a complex and difficult problem for home care policy. Several large jurisdictions have abandoned them or are in the process of doing so; yet it is uncertain whether others will follow suit and whether the independent provider route will remain a major alternative form of home care service. Administrative arrangements like those adopted by California (see Chapter 6) for centrally payrolling individual providers can solve some of the most pressing payment and payroll deduction problems, but ambiguities over legal status and debate over service quality remain. Because relatively extensive and therefore costly service is required for many home care clients, especially those with higher impairment levels, controlling cost per direct service hour will always remain a crucial issue for home care programs, in order for care at home to be financially viable. Administering agencies may feel at times caught between the Scylla of potential liability, quality problems, accusations of exploitation, and the other problems of the independent contractor system on the one hand, and the Charybdis of increased overhead costs. Like other important policy issues in home care, these issues can be better addressed with the benefit of feedback from a well-managed, integrated flow of both programmatic and fiscal information.

The themes described throughout Part I are exemplified by the five systems discussed in detail in Part II. These five systems—in Alameda County, Connecticut, Texas, Washington, and New York City—include a variety of alternative models for home care management. They present a range of ways in which information resources can be managed and integrated and appropriate controls implemented. While it will always be the case that each public jurisdiction constitutes a distinctive environment with a particular set of constraints, each also encounters similar administrative problems and can learn much from other existing systems.

PART II
Innovative Fiscal and Program Management Practices

6

Computer-Supported Case Assessment in Alameda County, California

Alameda County, California, has introduced microcomputers into decision making in its In-Home Supportive Services Program. The computers are used by social workers to help decide how many home care hours to award a client, as well as by program managers to assist in forecasting budgets and expenditures.

Computer assistance has reduced differences in the number of hours awarded to clients with similar characteristics. At the same time, the computerized system has created a data base from which information is produced to help in staff management and fiscal planning. This has improved management control over current-year expenditures as well as forecasting.

PROGRAM BACKGROUND

Alameda County is located in the San Francisco Bay Area. Its largest city is Oakland. The county's home care system, part of California's In-Home Supportive Services (IHSS) program, served approximately 5,500 frail elderly and disabled persons in fiscal year 1985. There was an average of nearly 4,000 active cases per month, with 92 new cases a month. By 1986 there were about 130 new cases a month.

In Alameda County, as in all California counties, a variety of domestic, food preparation/service/cleanup, and nonmedical personal services is available under the IHSS program. The range of services available in addition to daily care includes restaurant meal allowances for clients without food storage and preparation facilities; assistance by the provider for travel to medical or personal business appointments when the client is unable to make the trip without assistance; paramedical services when ordered by a licensed health care professional; yard hazard abatement; and protective supervision.

The average client received 15 hours of in-home service per week (65.9 hours per month), at an average cost of $225 per month in fiscal year 1985. (This increased to 73.2 hours per month by 1986, up to an average cost of $254 per month and 17 hours a week.) In all, this amounted to an expenditure of at least $11.4 million per year for client services. Revenue for client services is provided for in the state's General Fund budget, partially reimbursed through Federal Title XX Funds. IHSS service in Alameda County was managed and supervised by a staff of 60, which included social workers, supervisors, and clerks, at a total administrative cost of $2.6 million per year.

For a person to be eligible for services, he or she must be receiving or be eligible for SSI or California's State Supplementary Program (SSP). Where income exceeds the SSI/SSP eligibility (2 percent of the cases), the client must "spend down" his or her income to the SSI/SSP level before services are fully paid for by the program.

Each new client is assessed by an IHSS intake social worker. After the initial authorized level of services is set and service delivery begins, the client is transferred to a district social worker, who has a caseload of up to 160 cases. Eligibility is recertified by the district social worker once every 12 months or when changes occur in the individual's living or health situation.

Of the total client population served, approximately 76% were frail elderly over the age of 60. The balance were disabled and between the ages of 3 and 59 years. Of the total service population, 7% were defined as severely impaired and required 20 or more hours per week of specifically identified personal, nonmedical, meal, and paramedical services. The increase in hours and number of clients may be due to two factors: clients are living longer and are frailer; and/or the DRG system for hospital reimbursement may cause patients/clients to be sicker upon discharge from hospitals.

In California, a county may select one or a combination of three service delivery methods: care by county employees; purchase of service through county contracts with provider agencies; or purchase of service by the recipient from independent providers. In Alameda County the last method is used. Chore providers are hired by the client and were paid $3.58 per hour in 1985. A social worker may assist the client in recruiting, screening, and selecting a provider where the client needs the assistance.

California's IHSS home care program is state supervised but county administered. The legislature approves an annual budget for the service using state General Fund and federal Social Services Block Grant funds for the client service budget. The California State Department of Social Services supervises the program at the state level by allocating funds to each county, preparing and disseminating program regulations, interpreting applicable state and federal laws, providing technical assistance, and supervising the recipient-provider contractors. The Alameda County program was managed by an Adult Services Section Supervisor within the Human Services Department's Adult and Family Services Division.

All payments to clients or a client's provider are issued by a statewide payroll contractor, upon authorization by the county. Clients who are severely impaired may opt to receive their authorized level of funds in advance on the first day of each month, purchase required services during the month, and then turn in expenditure reports (time sheets) the following month. All other clients have their provider paid twice a month, after they have worked and submitted a time sheet. Of all authorized hours, 90 to 92% were claimed and paid in the same month in 1985. Time sheets are received by the county and checked for accuracy. Specific data are transmitted electronically to a central computer, which carries out the check-printing and mailing process.

DEVELOPMENT OF COMPUTER-ASSISTED ASSESSMENT

In 1977, Alameda County took part in a study by the Bay Area Welfare–University of California group, a consortium that involved five Bay Area welfare departments and a research group from the university. A principal concern of the study was that clients with similar needs were being awarded different numbers of service hours. These differences were believed to result in unnecessary increases in program costs. The study's aim was to document the set of rules that the participating counties were using to determine hours of homemaker or chore services awarded and to analyze the degree of equity associated with awards. The study found that awards to the "average" client were relatively inconsistent. The measure of consistency (the proportion of variance explained by case characteristics documented in the case record) ranged from 60 to 69% in different Bay Area counties and varied greatly in the different Alameda County district offices. On the basis of these findings, the study recommended a simplified uniform assessment form and use of a computer to display information on other workers' award decisions, as an approach to improve the equity of award decisions.

In response to this recommendation, the Alameda Department of Social Services joined with the University of California–Berkeley (UCB) School of Social Work in 1979 to undertake a three-year demonstration project. The Equity Project, as it became known, tested the hypothesis that, if social workers were given standard assessment forms, standard procedures, and a readily available history of previous assessments and allocations via a microcomputer, then more equitable decisions would result. Testing this hypothesis involved the design and implementation of, first, a standardized assessment form and guidelines and, second, an automated system for collecting the assessment information and predicting service-hour allocations based on the assessment data.

The development of the new system involved analyzing the process that social workers go through in assessing clients and awarding hours so that a computer program could be written to describe it. The process began with social workers discussing the factors that are most significant to their decisions on how many hours to award a client. A standardized assessment form was then developed to collect information on those factors in a framework that could be easily computerized. Because social workers use information on a client's functional limitations and social situation to evaluate the client's needs for the type of assistance that the program can provide, the assessment form was structured to describe the client's functioning and living situation. To standardize the functional evaluation, numerical values were assigned to the different functions so that the client's level of need for assistance could be scored.

Weights were assigned to the different functions, based upon a multiple regression analysis that determined each variable's contribution to explaining the awards received by clients. The computer multiplies each functional assessment score by its assigned weight, totals the products, and produces an eligibility index for each client. The computer then displays a "predicted award" for the client currently being assessed, based on the average award for similar cases previously assessed.

Design, testing, and refinement of the computer-assisted assessment was for the most part completed in the first two years of the demonstration project. In addition to the conceptual design of the system, another major task undertaken was the creation of an initial data base that the computer could draw on to make its predictions. Researchers from UCB coded several thousand existing and prior cases and calculated their hour awards using the county's time-per-task guidelines and eligibility indexes. The demonstration sustained the initial hypothesis for the research effort, finding that the consistency of workers' allocation decisions did indeed improve with use of the standard assessment forms and procedures—including instant feedback, via the microcomputer, of information on previous allocations to similar cases. The consistency measure in Alameda County now ranges from 87 to 90 percent.

MAKING HOUR AWARDS USING THE COMPUTER

The process of allocating service hours using the computer differs from other assessment and allocation processes in an important way: Workers must put their assessment information into the computer and then take the computer predictions into account in their award decisions. The process is as follows:

1. The social worker makes a home visit and, via question and observation, assesses and scores the client's functioning level according to the assessment guidelines. The worker notes on a form the services needed by the client and assesses and records the extent of existing help from other persons or agencies, under four major service categories.

2. The social worker returns to the office and enters the assessment information into the computer. The worker then receives from the computer predictions on the number of hours needed for domestic, meal, and personal services; the total predicted number of weekly hours; and whether or not the client is classifiable as severely impaired. It also provides an eligibility index score.

3. The social worker recommends a service-hour award. This involves checking on the assessment form those tasks for which client hours will be awarded and proposing the number of hours to be awarded under various service categories (such as domestic, meal, personal, and other). This determination is expected to be made on the basis of the prediction and on special client circumstances. Hours for each discrete task within general service categories need not be calculated or reported. If the total proposed award for domestic, meal, and personal services is significantly different from the computer-predicted total of these categories, the worker is required to comment on the reason for the differences on the assessment form. Commonly occurring comments (such as flat-rate case, client independence, fair hearing decision) have already been preprinted on the form. To enable workers to anticipate when comments will be requested, the computer displays both the predicted award and the expected range of award variation for each case. The service plan is then reviewed and approved by the supervisor or section supervisor.

4. The social worker then enters the award information into the computer. Depending upon when the worker is prepared to make his or her award decision, the award information may be entered immediately or after discussing the equity predictions with the supervisor. Award information may be separately entered later by reentering the worker

and client numbers and indicating that the assessment information has already been entered. If previously entered award information is changed after the supervisory discussion, the changed award may be entered into the computer in the same way. In practice the award data are most often entered before supervisory approval and changed later if necessary.

5. The social worker discusses the recommended award with the client, reaches an agreement, and formally notifies the client of the award via a Notice of Action letter.

PROGRAM IMPACT

The development and implementation of the computer-assisted award system have been seen in Alameda County as methods for improving the equitable assignment of service hours to clients rather than as ways of controlling program costs. Nonetheless, the revamped assessment and eligibility index system contains elements that the management in Alameda County sees as being tied in with and of benefit to the fiscal management of In-Home Supportive Services. Certainly, to the extent that increasing the equity of hour allocations keeps down the number of service hours awarded, the new system directly contributes to cost containment, because authorization of service hours is the primary determinant of program costs. It would be misleading, however, to claim that the system is a method for containing costs. Just as it may decrease the number of hours awarded to some clients, it may increase the hours awarded to others and thereby add to program costs.

One of the system's attributes is its capacity to improve management of the allocation process and thus indirectly of resource allocation. The design of the computer-assisted system builds allocation policies into the process of making award decisions. The computer is programmed to predict hour awards on the basis of previous authorizations, which in turn reflect established allocation policies and rules. This is coupled with a process that requires that deviations from predictions receive additional explanation and documentation. In combination, these two factors tend to assure that the key allocation policies are consistently applied in relation to every award decision, although the actual award may, with justification, vary from the rules.

In practice, the Alameda computerized system has decreased paperwork and the average time required to review most case awards. It has also focused attention on cases that differ from the norm. To assure consistent application of allocation rules in a noncomputerized system entails much closer review and supervision of individual hour award decisions. The noncomputerized system that had previously operated in Alameda County relied on judgmental decisions and seemed more open to arguments between supervisors and social workers over award decisions. The computerized system has given the worker and the supervisor an agreed-upon data base. This has greatly reduced stress associated with decision making when the recommended award is within the norm.

Another area where the system has yielded improvements has been that of monitoring and quality control. Using the award data in its files, the computer can generate periodic reports on an individual worker's or a supervisory unit's record of award decisions. These reports display both graphically and numerically how the cases assessed measure up to predicted awards. The reports are given to individual workers and supervisors so that they can see how their decisions compare to the norm. This helps workers and managers to review the pattern of their decisions and identify where and why their behavior may be different. Where reasons for the difference are the misapplication or misinterpretation of assessment and allocation policies, this can be corrected. Alameda County does not expect complete conformity with predicted awards. Full consistency might indicate that workers are not exercising professional judgment in applying allocation rules.

Apart from introducing the computer into the social worker's life, the redesigned assessment process has reduced the time required to assess a client's need. Formerly, home visits took from 1.5 to 2 hours; now they take 30 to 45 minutes. The system has also cut the time formerly spent on time-per-task calculations. The computer calculates a predicted award in a matter of seconds.

For the client the system has meant more equitable service hour awards. This has reduced the number of client complaints and appeals because clients and client advocates understand the basis for awarding hours.

BUDGET FORECASTING

Once they had developed a computerized assessment and award data base, the IHSS program managers saw the opportunity to use the data to improve their budget planning and expenditure forecasting capacity. Under contract with the same University of California–Berkeley staff that developed the assessment program, and assisted by funds from the Home Care Fiscal Management Project, Alameda County developed a budget program that links the assessment data base with the monthly expenditure and caseload data from the automated payroll contractor.

The budget program enables the program manager to use actual caseload data to project the impact that changes in program policy, wage and tax rates, caseload, law, and/or regulations will have on expenditures. This allows the manager to predict whether or not such changes will result in future expenditures exceeding the fixed budget allocation for client services. When it can be predicted that such changes will result in future expenditures exceeding the budget, the computer can consider the various corrective options and help calculate for the program manager what the cost savings might be and how the changes might impact the caseload.

The following example may help illustrate how the program is used for forecasting. Suppose that a new state regulation is approved in September which increases the maximum domestic service award from four to five hours per week. The change is to go into effect January 1. The program manager needs to know how this change is going to affect the budget, which has already been fixed for the fiscal year that runs from July 1 to June 30. The impact of the regulatory change depends on two things: the number of clients affected and when the change goes into effect. Depending on the client's scheduled reassessment date, the change might go into effect January 1, in which case the increased cost would affect six months of the fiscal year; or it might go into effect April 1, in which case the increase would affect only three months.

Using the budget program, the computer tells the program manager in a few seconds how many cases are presently at the maximum domestic service award and how many of these are up for reassessment between January and June. The manager can then use the program to calculate, on the basis of the reassessment dates of the affected cases, what the service cost increase will be if the assumption is made that all the reassessed cases will be awarded the increase to the new maximum of five domestic service hours per week. If the calculated cost increase fits within the service budget, no further forecasting is required. However, if the budget program's calculations indicate that the universal increase of those at the current maximum will result in over-expending the service budget, the manager has to consider different policies that may be used to govern the implementation of the new rule. The budget program can calculate the cost increases that would arise under different conditions. The manager can use the budget program to calculate what the cost increase would be if it is assumed that 75 percent, rather than 100 percent, of reassessments are awarded the increase, or if the increase is restricted to cases above a certain eligibility index score.

In less than five minutes the program manager can come up with data on the impact of the policy change on the service budget as well as the impact that various implementation options will have on both the budget and caseload. Thus, the computerized assessment and award data base, when linked to the budgeting process, has the clear benefit of enabling cost projections to be made on the basis of actual caseload information.

POTENTIAL FOR REPLICATION

In order to replicate Alameda County's computer-assisted service-hour allocation system at other relocations, some preconditions would need to be met. An obvious precondition is purchasing or getting use of microcomputers. Alameda County was using the Apple II Plus in 1986, but other widely used microcomputers would also be suitable. A printer is also required to produce the necessary reports.

In addition to the computer hardware, software is needed and a data base for predicting hour allocations has to be in place. Copies of Alameda's program diskettes and instruction booklets are available from the County Social Service Agency. However, depending upon local variations in the methods and rules regarding allocation of service hours, the Alameda program might need to be adapted. Alameda County staff believe that the adaptation could be made by any programmer with a math and computer science background.

Another precondition in California was getting approval from the state to waive mandated time-per-task guidelines. While these were the basis for computerized hour allocations, equity is judged on the overall hour award, thereby departing from strict adherence to time-per-task. Other sites may or may not require such legislative or regulatory waivers.

Alameda's system has several selling points. Program managers benefit from the reports that the data base generates. The reports provide feedback on workers' award practices and on how well each unit's workers assess client needs. The data base provides information that facilitates budget forecasting decisions, including those on how reductions in expenditures can be achieved in an orderly fashion when required.

When originally proposed and introduced, the system did encounter some opposition. The social workers' union opposed it, fearing it would reduce jobs and be used for negative personnel actions. There was also a fear of computers on the part of most staff and fear of their intrusion into the confines of the social workers' professional assessment. Over time, these concerns have eased. In part, this was achieved because the approach used to implement the computer-assisted allocation system was incremental. The shift to the new system began with a small group of social workers who volunteered for the job, not by mandating it as the sole assessment methodology. As other social workers observed how the system worked and how easy it was to use, they began to adopt it. Fear of machines and union opposition slowly disappeared. Fears about intrusion into the confines of the professional role have been addressed by encouraging staff to make their own final award decisions and to use the predicted award solely as the peer-developed guideline that it is.

CONCLUSION

By 1986, Alameda County's microcomputer-based system had been in successful operation for several years and information on the project had been widely disseminated through the Home Care Fiscal Management Project's workshops and fiscal report. During that year, the State of California decided to mandate statewide implementation of the system, issued an administrative letter requiring implementation in 1987, and formed an advisory group to assist it in developing the plan for introducing the system. This important action by California (with a home care caseload of 117,000 in 1986) represents significant progress in the integrated and systematic use of information systems to advance the goals of home care management—particularly, in this case, the goal of attaining comparable treatment of similarly situated clients. Integrating client characteristics data with fiscal and other data also means that trends in the program can be much more effectively monitored and projected.

7

Performance-Based Contracting in Connecticut

In 1975 the Connecticut Department on Aging decided that community-based care for the very frail elderly could best be achieved by effectively coordinating the delivery of a wide range of social and health services. For this purpose the department decided that each client should have an individual care plan designed to meet his or her specific needs. To obtain the resources needed to implement these care plans, it would also be desirable to tap multiple funding sources.

Based on these requirements and in light of its earlier experience with TRIAGE, a pioneering demonstration of case management in Connecticut, the Department on Aging adopted a case management model for its Promotion of Independent Living program. However, the model that was adopted differed from previous programs. The case manager's responsibility included not only needs assessment and care planning for the delivery of department-funded services, but also the coordination of other services and funding sources. The purpose of comprehensive case management was to ensure that the total care plan was adequate to meet the program's goal of maintaining individuals in the community.

Since the budget under the department's control was inadequate to meet the needs of all the elderly who were potentially eligible, the effective use of outside resources was critical, not only to insure adequate care plans but also to maximize the number of people the Promotion of Independent Living program could serve. The department therefore stipulated that its own funds could be used only after the case managers had tapped all available outside resources.

To measure the extent to which case management maximized the effectiveness of the program, the department applied performance-based contracting to the Promotion of Independent Living program. This practice provided accountability for program funds, together with the leveraging of outside resources by establishing performance standards in the case management contract.

PROGRAM BACKGROUND

The goal of Connecticut's Promotion of Independent Living program is to prevent the premature and/or inappropriate institutionalization of elderly clients. In order to bring together the most appropriate package of services for a client, there is a single entry point to the program. This entry point is a case management agency, which is responsible for eligibility, assessment, development of care plans, procuring and coordinating services for the client, and monitoring client progress. As conceived of by the Department on Aging, the single entry point serves two purposes. One is to bring together the most appropriate mix of social and medical services on behalf of the client. The other is to have a single point of accountability for the cost and appropriateness of the total service package.

Until 1986 the program was operated statewide by Connecticut Community Care, Inc. (CCCI), the successor agency to TRI-AGE, under a contract with the Department on Aging. CCCI both provides case management services and administers the departmental funds budgeted for purchasing services for clients. For fiscal year 1987, the department went to a competitive procurement process.

Case management agencies are licensed by the Connecticut

Department of Health, as coordination, assessment, and monitoring (CAM) agencies. As such the services a CAM agency can provide directly are limited to assessment, care planning, counseling, and monitoring. Other direct services must be obtained from outside agencies.

CAM agencies obtain services for clients through contracts with local providers, who may be nonprofit or proprietary agencies or, in some instances, private individuals. Each contract specifies a unit cost for each service the agency offers. Specific services are purchased as needed through service orders for the individual client. In this way the CAM agency retains control over the type and amount of service ordered and the choice of provider for each client. By shopping among local providers, the CAM agency is able to obtain the most appropriate service for a specific client at the best price.

In Connecticut, all home health care rates for all state clients are set by the Commission on Hospitals and Health Care. Rates for homemaker, chore service, companion, and adult day care agencies are negotiated with each provider individually.

The Promotion of Independent Living program was budgeted at $4.8 million in fiscal year 1984. Thirty-five percent of the funds were from the Social Services Block Grant and 65 percent from the state's general fund. In fiscal year 1984 the program served an average of 2,740 cases a month. The client population's average age was 79.2 years, with an average annual income of $4,634. Nearly 75% of all clients were women, 55% were widowed, and 47% lived alone. With respect to the client population's eligibility for other programs, 86% had Medicare supplementary medical insurance, 75% were eligible for Title 20 services, and 18% were eligible for Medicaid.

To qualify as eligible for Promotion of Independent Living services, an individual must be

- A resident of Connecticut
- 60 years of age or older
- Either inappropriately institutionalized or at risk of inappropriate institutionalization, as determined by a comprehensive assessment process
- In need of case management services

Elderly persons with incomes at or below 150 percent of the poverty level are eligible for services at no cost. Those with incomes between 150 and 200 percent of the poverty level are required to share in the cost of their purchased services on a sliding scale. Priority is given to individuals eligible for Supplemental Security Income, State Supplemental Assistance, or Medicaid, as well as to low-income elderly, minority elderly, and individuals who are inappropriately institutionalized.

At the state level, the Promotion of Independent Living program is the responsibility of the Commissioner on Aging and the Research and Programs Development Division. Day-to-day operations are handled by one program manager, with the aid of the department's fiscal office (which processes financial reports) and the planning staff (which assists with matters of policy and data evaluation).

PROGRAM MODEL

In order to understand the fiscal management practices applied to the Promotion of Independent Living program, it is first necessary to understand the case management model on which it operates. The basic steps of the case management approach are

1. Determining program eligibility
2. Providing a comprehensive assessment of the client's needs
3. Developing a care plan to address those needs
4. Assisting clients in obtaining services called for in the plan
5. Monitoring the appropriateness of the plan over time

Two features distinguish Connecticut's Promotion of Independent Living program from many others. One is the way in which control over eligibility determination, care planning, and financial management is contracted to a nonprofit agency. The other feature that distinguishes Connecticut's program model is the fact that it is aimed at coordinating multiple services funded through a variety of sources. The effect of this is that assisting clients in obtaining services is not an automatic matter of authorizing the purchase or provision of service from program funds. Instead, it is a process of trying to build comprehensive care plans and getting access to nonprogram dollars and resources. The outside resources that may be available to a client might include other governmental programs such as Medicare, Medicaid, or adult social services; or nongovernmental supports such as the client's family or community agencies. The case manager only uses departmental funds to procure services when there is a gap in the care plan that cannot be bridged with other funds. The effect of this is that, while a client may receive a package of home care services, the single service for which the Promotion of Independent Living program may pay may be case management.

A program of this kind places demands on the fiscal management system that are more complex than they would be under a simpler program model. In addition to tracking expenditures, assuring their correctness and validity, and providing an audit trail, the fiscal management system provides a means for the department (1) to retain full knowledge and effective control over the ongoing operations of the program and (2) to track the contractor's effectiveness in leveraging outside resources.

DEVELOPMENT OF PERFORMANCE-BASED CONTRACTING

The Department on Aging adopted the practice of performance-based contracting in its 1983 contract with CCCI. The contract establishes performance goals and targets that enable the state to gauge performance against the goal of serving the greatest number of clients possible while limiting the department's cost per client.

Adoption of the performance-based contracting method was a natural outgrowth of the development of performance-oriented management. This management method itself evolved from the reporting and monitoring systems that came into play shortly after the start of the Promotion of Independent Living program in 1976-1977. From its earliest days the reporting system tracked administrative and service costs, cost per client, commitments of service dollars, clients served, and services provided. Initially, the object of collecting this information was to assist in managing the program's finances and operations so as to avoid the overcommitment of resources that had occurred early in the program's history.

Prior to 1981 the program was operated by the state's five Area Agencies on Aging. The reporting system at this stage was basically a manual effort to obtain data on performance that the state could use for its planning and management of the program.

At the state agency level the system was partially automated. When operation of the Promotion of Independent Living program was shifted to Connecticut Community Care in 1981, the reporting system went through another stage of development. CCCI offered a vastly improved management capacity and a large computer capable of handling both its day-to-day management needs and the department's reporting requirements. In light of this, the Department on Aging reviewed existing requirements for performance data and adapted them to reflect the data collection and processing capacity of CCCI's automated management information systems. The result was that the new reporting requirements generated a series of reports in proper accounting format that were accurate and sophisticated enough for CCCI management and the Department on Aging to use for monitoring performance and operations.

Incorporating performance goals into CCCI's contract was a natural step in the development of the program. What it added to the previous reporting system was accountability for performance by (1) setting expectations at the beginning of the contract period, for which CCCI was held accountable; and (2) linking CCCI's bimonthly payment to satisfactory performance, as measured by the goals and indicators. The state's program manager is now able to monitor progress toward meeting performance goals, through a series of reports required at regular intervals under the terms of the contracts.

In administering the contract, the Department on Aging practices management by exception, intervening only when the contractor deviates significantly from the expectations established in the contract. In a continuous monitoring system such as the one the department employs, the test of significant deviation is based on projection to determine if deviations from the program plan threaten the contractor's ability to meet its annual goals. Therefore, a 5% variance at the end of the first quarter is far less significant than the same variance would be if it occurred at the end of the third quarter. If the department determines that a contractor has deviated from the program plan, the first step in the oversight process is to request corrective action. The request may be in the form of a phone call or a written request. If a CAM agency fails to comply with a request or give a satisfactory explanation why it has not done so within 30 days, the department may withhold funds. The ultimate sanction is that the department may cancel the contract for any reason, upon 90 days' notice.

While sanctions exist, the purpose of the performance goals and the monitoring system is to maximize the service delivered to clients. The goal of the monitoring process is therefore corrective action, with no need for sanctions. The performance measures used in the system are essentially the same ones used by the department to monitor the program and the same measures CCCI used to obtain management information. Therefore, the transition to performance-based contracting did not require many changes in operational or data gathering procedures.

The performance-based contract has had no direct impact on service providers because services are obtained through purchase of service contracts based on fixed rates and individual service orders. However, there is an indirect impact because cost effectiveness is one of the measures used to evaluate performance; thus, attaining the established goals within a fixed budget encourages cost containment. Cost becomes a factor in deciding which provider agency's services will be ordered and, when choices exist, which service will be chosen. Connecticut has a highly competitive home care delivery system. Services may be available from one or more public or nonprofit agencies and from as many as five proprietary agencies in any part of the state. In addition, the case manager can sometimes select from a variety of options such as homemaker services, adult day care, companions, and meals on wheels in preparing an individual's plan of care. The existence of these options is an important factor in making performance goals a meaningful activity.

MEASURING PROGRAM PERFORMANCE

The way in which the Connecticut Department on Aging has applied performance-based contracting enables it to measure several aspects of the operation of the Promotion of Independent Living program. When considered together, the different measurements enable the department and its subcontractor CAM agencies to assess how effective a job they are doing at serving the greatest number of clients possible by containing the department's cost per client.

Goals have been established for five main areas of the operation of Promotion of Independent Living. These include: individuals served; services provided; program income and third party funding; financial leveraging; and client cost data. For each area, several performance indicators are defined. For example, in the program income and third party funding area, indicators include the amount of Medicare and Medicaid funding secured, and client and family payments. In the client cost area, one measure is the cost per unduplicated client per year, a measure which varies with the average duration of service, while another is the cost per average monthly client per year. In the financial leveraging area, indicators include administrative cost and case management (CAM) cost, both as a percentage of total costs. The latter two sets of indicators are calculated two ways: inclusive and exclusive of nondepartmentally funded services secured for clients. This approach focuses management attention on leveraging the maximum possible nondepartmentally funded services.

The exact goals are set by the department on the basis of its knowledge of CAM agencies' capabilities and historical data. They are subject to negotiation as part of the contract process. Because the performance goals are linked to the contract budget, it is important to recognize, in establishing goals, that there are factors that may have an impact on the budget but are outside program control. Some flexibility must be allowed, in order to take such things into account. For example, in Connecticut, provider rates have a tremendous impact on cost and cost per client but are set by other state agencies based on independent cost data. Since rate changes can take effect in the middle of the program year, unanticipated major rate changes can seriously affect the program's ability to meet its goals. Similarly, the program's ability to meet its goals for leveraging outside resources depends on the continued availability of those resources. In 1983 Connecticut's efforts in this area were seriously hampered by federal efforts to tighten utilization control screens for Medicare and by a virtual cutoff of services funded through a major state social services program. In 1985 continued federal efforts to tighten Medicare both reduced the availability of Medicare funding and had an impact on rates for non–Medicare patients.

Major changes in the availability of third-party resources are regularly reported to the department (or by the department to the CAM agency), and their potential impact on the CAM agency's ability to meet its goals is projected. Since the availability of third-party resources is almost always beyond the control of the contractor, the CAM agency is not penalized when such changes occur.

Once the contract has been negotiated and the performance targets set, the CAM agency submits reports on a monthly and quarterly basis to the department's program manager. Monthly reports include an income and expense statement, which contains monthly and year-to-date data and variances from the program's spending plan; a monthly caseload report which shows both current and year-to-date caseloads as well as intake and discharge activity by region; a monthly activity report which details activity levels by case management function; and a client census and purchased service report, which shows clients by payment status and relates clients and service costs in creating a display of cost-per-client trends. One quarterly report details client characteristics, while another lists cost per client by funding source and as an overall total. Each of these reports contains data used in the management of the program as well as information that can be used to measure how well the CAM agency is succeeding in meeting its performance goals.

The income and expense statement, and especially the information on year-to-date variances that it contains, relates to the fundamental requirement that the provider remain within the spending limits fixed in the contract. The monthly caseload report relates directly to the first performance indicator, the number of individuals served. The monthly activity report is tied to the second performance indicator, services provided. The client census and purchased service report provides information on client costs and is one of the most important management tools for projecting trends in average monthly cost.

The quarterly report on cost per client, broken down by funding source, summarizes both the project's success in obtaining third-party funding and the contractor's performance in terms of total cost per client from all funding sources, one of the client cost indicators. Finally, the quarterly report of client characteristics, along with quality assurance reviews, is a measure of how well the CAM agency targets its program toward the population it is intended to serve.

In addition to reviewing each of these reports individually, the department reviews them as a group, to insure that performance meets expectations. Staying within budget targets is only satisfactory if the effort serves an appropriate number of clients from the target population. Success in leveraging outside resources is only a desirable outcome if it can be achieved while remaining

**TABLE 7-1 Promotion-of-Independent-Living Clients
Categorized by Funding Source**

Funding source	Number of clients	Percentage of total clients
Program funds only	242	9.2
Program funds and family contributions	789	29.9
Third-party funding only (Title XVIII, XIX, III B&C, private foundations, and other)	412	15.6
Third-party & family contributions	364	13.8
Program, Title III third-party, family contributions	828	31.4
TOTAL	2,635	99.9

within the approved budget and while providing needed services to appropriate clients.

At the provider level, collection and processing of performance data requires input from the agency's executive and deputy directors, its accountant, its data systems supervisor, and its regional office staffs. However, since much of the information collected is used in the day-to-day administration of the provider agency, obtaining it does not represent an exceptional burden generated by performance-based contracting itself.

Case management's success in extending funds available through the Promotion of Independent Living program can be seen from performance targets in the contract. The average monthly caseload in fiscal year 1983 increased by 240, and the average value of services per client per year increased by some $1,300. The program cost element that most benefits from leveraging is purchased services. This is because the department's funds buy only 35 percent of all services, but they pay for over 90 percent of administration and case management cost. Thus, in the context of the *total* of funded and leveraged costs, the Promotion of Independent Living program pays 48% of all costs. This indicates a major extension of the program's budgeted capacity. The total leveraged program budget is some $10 million, of which the department's share is $4.8 million.

To analyze performance in leveraging nonprogram dollars from a different perspective, Connecticut categorized clients in November 1983, according to the sources that were funding their services. The results are shown in Table 7-1.

The most obvious impact of leveraging is that it substantially increases the number of clients the program can serve. Clients also benefit when leveraging makes possible more extensive care plans than the program might otherwise be able to provide. Another indirect benefit of the practice is that many families are encouraged to continue taking an active interest in the client's well-being, whereas they might otherwise feel overwhelmed by the burden of caring of their elderly relatives and abandon them altogether.

Critics of the Connecticut model may contend that leveraging outside resources contains costs only within the parameters of the department's budget. Proponents of leveraging through case management might argue that focusing on the cost-shifting effects of comprehensive care planning loses sight of the primary goals of the program and their cost implications. As provided in Connecticut, community-based care is less costly than institutional care. If coordinated care planning makes it possible to maintain an individual in the home, it costs far less under the program guidelines than it would if the individual were institutionalized. Leveraging makes it possible to produce comprehensive care plans in an environment where no single funding source might be able to support the full range of services needed. Leveraging also allows more clients at risk of institutionalization to be served, thus providing more opportunities for avoiding institutionalization and reducing costs. Finally, case management provides a means of coordinating several funding sources and providers and reducing service duplication and excess care costs.

LINKAGES TO FISCAL MANAGEMENT

Performance-based contracting is itself a fiscal management system that extends from budgeting and program planning through accounting and reporting and, ultimately, through program evaluation. A major advantage of performance-based contracting, in comparison with other fiscal management systems, is that it is tied to the service delivery system at every stage of the administrative management process.

Leveraging is incorporated into the financial management process through program budgeting. Under program budgeting all funding sources are taken into account in the development of the service targets and the program's staffing and management plan. Once the program budget and performance-based contracts are in place, information gathering and reporting requirements associated with them become regular fiscal management tools of the program; the program's accounting systems are designed to meet these system needs. Under program budgeting, cost allocation systems and program audits assume greater importance than they might otherwise, since charges must be accurately allocated to each funding source and program (if the agency has more than one). However, since leveraged resources are by definition outside the accounting control of the program, they are not subject to audit. They must therefore be monitored as part of the program evaluation process.

POTENTIAL FOR REPLICATION

Performance-based contracting and leveraging outside resources can be implemented separately or as part of an overall management plan. Since the potential applications of the two processes and the preconditions for applying them differ, it may be easier to consider their potential for replication separately.

Replication of Performance-Based Contracting

Before a program can be tied to expectations or standards for performance, a system for measuring performance must be developed. Such a system should include a clear statement of goals, measures of effectiveness, and procedures for record keeping, reporting, and monitoring. A performance measurements system can be developed for either a contract program or an in-house operation. For full effectiveness, there must be a strong fiscal and data management capacity at both the state agency and the provider levels.

The administering agency should be very careful to insure that the goals and expectations included in a performance-based contract are realistic. If the contractor cannot be reasonably expected to meet the administering agency's expectations concerning service delivery, record keeping, reporting, and program management, the practice cannot be implemented. Similarly, if the service goals are set too high, the program may be doomed to failure.

The administering agency must recognize that there is a cost in time and effort that goes into maintaining the administrative systems associated with performance monitoring and evaluation. Therefore, the program must be large enough to justify the expense involved. Any add-on costs can be minimized if the performance measurement system is designed to meet the operation needs of the program as well as the monitoring requirements of the administering agency.

As with any other program, there should be expectations for improvement over time in the operation of the program. Performance measurement can be useful in a variety of ways, including increasing the amount of service delivered to clients, improving the targeting of a program, or establishing a means of comparing contract agencies providing like services under similar conditions. It is important to have a clear idea of what the system is expected to accomplish before a project is undertaken, to insure that the system is properly designed and that its outputs have a benefit to the agency.

Finally, since performance-based contracting is based on holding the provider accountable in terms of meeting predefined goals, it is important to know enough about both the goals and the environment in which the program operates to determine which factors the contractor can control and which are beyond the contractor's ability to influence. A home care contractor cannot control changes in Medicare policy at the federal level; thus, the case management agency cannot be held responsible for the impact of such changes on its progress in achieving performance targets.

The most likely source of opposition to the introduction of a performance-based contracting system may be provider agencies that are accountable for the money they receive. To some extent this may be unavoidable, since performance evaluation implies that there will be new sanctions if the provider fails to meet expectations. However, this may be minimized if the program is adequately designed and carefully explained.

Potential contractors should be introduced to the concept in an orderly fashion. Performance measurement should be in place before performance-based contracting is attempted.

Performance goals should be realistic if the administering agency hopes to gain provider acceptance. Similarly, there should be a realistic and workable plan for implementing the system, including establishing program goals, developing ac-

counting systems, and fulfilling reporting requirements. If contractors are presented with what appears to be an impossible
task, they will resist it. Since the concepts of performance measurement are likely to be new to many contractors, the administering agency should be prepared to provide substantial technical assistance during the development phase.

Performance monitoring and evaluation can substantially improve the management of a home care program. Providers can
be offered the prospect of improved management and better
program performance as an inducement for cooperating in the
implementation of performance management systems.

There may be pitfalls, too. One potential mistake can be to
attempt to adopt performance-based contracting without adequate advance planning. Problems also may arise if the project is
undertaken without ensuring that adequate administrative resources are available at both the state and local levels. At the state
level, performance-based contracting involves program planning, organization and management, and strong financial administration skills. Since many of the concepts involved are similar
to those used to manage programs in private industry, a state
agency might look to graduates of business administration programs for the skills required.

Another potential danger in developing a performance-based
contracting system is that the designers may lose sight of the
primary purpose of the program. The primary purpose of Connecticut's home care program is to provide an efficient and effective network of community-based long-term care for the elderly. Appropriate measures of program performance could
therefore include the number of clients maintained in their own
homes, measures of cost compared to other institutional or community-based long-term care programs, or measures of the extent to which the provider is serving the program's target population. Inappropriate measures might be ones that focus on staff
activity or service volume without determining that individuals
are being maintained in the community or that the cost per client
compares favorably with other alternatives. Similarly, leveraging is a useful way of extending the limited resources of a home
care program, but the amount of money leveraged says nothing
about the overall cost of care or the appropriateness of care
plans.

Replication of Leveraging Third-Party Resources

A precondition for leveraging is adopting the concept of comprehensive case management for assessment and care planning. Leveraging involves exploring a range of funding sources which support an array of services designed to meet a variety of needs. The purpose of this activity is to build comprehensive care plans. If the program were to involve only the provision of a single service to meet a narrowly defined need, seeking outside resources might more properly be termed cost shifting or cost sharing.

The effective coordination of outside funding sources adds to the care planning process complexity; therefore, the case management staff need to have broader qualifications and presumably a higher level of training than the typical caseworker.

Any program that proposes to adopt leveraging as a practice should also have a regulation, a contractual requirement, or a policy statement that incorporates leveraging into the operation program. If a home care program is designated as an entitlement, there is no justification for requesting the participation of third-party payers. In addition, the program is likely to be stymied by "payer of last resort" clauses in the program guidelines of their funding sources.

While leveraging can be an effective means of supplementing program funds, the agency should have a pool of funds under its direct control with which to purchase services. Otherwise, there is no guarantee that third-party funds will be sufficient to develop comprehensive care plans that meet client needs and achieve the goals of the program. At the same time, the availability of program funds may act as an incentive for other funding sources to cooperate in the care planning process.

Successful implementation of a policy on the use of third-party funds may be heavily dependent upon both the skill of the case managers and having an assessment tool that captures the data the case managers need in order to identify possible outside resources and initiate applications. Therefore, training case managers is essential. Case managers who work best in the community are those who are adept at assessing client and family needs and resources. They should also be knowledgeable about all of the supports within the community and well versed in how the social welfare system can be made to work for the benefit of their clients. Training of case managers should also emphasize the importance of interdisciplinary teamwork. Social workers and nurses will need a broad range of skills in assessing client needs and arranging appropriate care plans, working with the family to develop an informal support network, and gaining access to alternative funding sources.

An assessment tool that can be used to evaluate a case management system should be designed with the information needs of other funding sources in mind. This implies a thorough knowledge of the eligibility requirements of the other funding sources and of the information that needs to be supplied when an application for third-party funding is prepared. If leveraging is to be formally incorporated into a program plan or performance-based contract, it will be necessary to keep records on outside funds leveraged. Once baseline data have been gathered, targets can be set and eventually formal leveraging goals can be established.

A policy of leveraging has a basic financial appeal in that it can be used to extend program resources and increase services to the target population. In addition, leveraging can sometimes make it possible to assemble care plans that might otherwise involve services not allowable through program funding sources. This may in turn mean the difference to a client between institutionalization and remaining in the community.

One of the main difficulties in integrating leveraging into a home care program is that most case managers are nurses or social workers, and they may believe that their talents are best utilized in needs assessment counseling rather than case management. Care must therefore be taken in the hiring, training, and supervision of case managers. Inadequately trained case managers constitute perhaps the greatest potential pitfall to a program that includes leveraging. Other potential difficulties include the possibility that care plans that include leveraged funds may be excessively costly, regardless of fund source, or that case managers may neglect other aspects of case management while pursuing outside resources. Preventing these problems is largely a management and supervisory function. The best way to insure that they do not occur is to focus on the agency's program goal: maintaining individuals in the community.

8

System-Based Contracting in Texas

The Texas Department of Human Services has developed a systematic approach to its contracts that increases the state's control over both the cost and quality of services. The comprehensive process goes beyond performance-based contracting to consider the entire life of a contracted service, from service definition to procurement, contract monitoring, and, where necessary, contract termination. The Texas system is also a good illustration of how a fiscal management system can be integrated with service management. This is accomplished by developing service and fiscal control systems that are essentially mirror images of each other. Key steps in both processes are service authorization, delivery, and payment so that, with the flat-rate system used to reimburse vendors, Texas can reconcile hours authorized and delivered with hours billed. The post-audit process is also greatly simplified because the necessary paper trail is created at the time of service delivery. In addition, with interdependent service and fiscal control, discrepancies such as those between authorized and actual initiation dates or service levels are almost wholly eliminated. The key to this integrated system is the statewide use of common source-control personnel and auditors.

PROGRAM BACKGROUND

In the late 1970s the Texas Department of Human Services (DHS) operated three Title XX-funded in-home programs. All served the same population, but there was wide variation in rates, service quality, availability, provider selection, and management. Each program had its own standards; the number of standards of the three programs totaled more than 130. This led to much confusion in the field about what was expected of a contractor. Compliance with program standards was very low. Contractors were paid on a cost reimbursement basis with a unit-rate ceiling, greatly complicating budget management and leading to numerous audit exceptions.

As the Texas Legislature began to place more emphasis on community-based care, the Texas DHS recognized that it was necessary for the delivery of home care services to be improved and made more consistent across the state. To accomplish this task, the department undertook to redesign its in-home program. The goal of redesigning was to develop a program of consistent quality and quantity across the state, but one that was still flexible enough to meet unique local needs. In early stages of the redesigning, both central and local office staffs agreed that any requirements placed on local staff or contractors must have a clearly stated purpose and must ultimately result in improved services to clients. In addition, programs were to be simple to administer and inexpensive.

To accomplish these goals, the staff developed a new contracting practice that uses a systems approach. This approach considers the entire life of a contracted service, from initial service definition to contract completion or cancellation. It integrates both service delivery and fiscal expectations and links budgeting, accounting, auditing, and performance measurement systems, through the use of common source documents. The resulting system gives the Texas DHS considerable control over both the cost and quality of in-home services.

In-home services in Texas are delivered through two programs: Family Care and Primary Home Care. Family Care is funded through the Social Services Block Grant (formerly Title

XX) and state general revenue funds. Primary Home Care, a Title XIX service, is funded by state-matched Medicaid funds. Both programs provide personal care, housekeeping, and escort services. In addition, nurse supervision and physician orders are required for services funded through the Primary Home Care program.

Texas DHS administers the in-home services program through 10 state regional offices that contract with local home health agencies according to statewide policies and procedures. In fiscal year 1985, approximately $49 million was spent on the Family Care program, which served more than 22,600 clients a month. The Primary Home Care program served over 20,000 clients a month at an annual cost of over $70 million. The provider base for in-home services includes sole proprietorships, public agencies, and nonprofit and for-profit agencies.

All home care clients enter the delivery system through Texas DHS's staff of case managers and nurses. This locally based staff determines eligibility and sets the amount (up to a maximum of 20 service hours per week in Family Care and 30 in Primary Home Care) and type of service the client will receive. They then send to a contractor an authorization to initiate service. This process gives the department complete control over service utilization. By monitoring the client at least every 180 days, the case manager is able to make adjustments in the service plan to meet a client's changing needs.

Family Care services include meal preparation and escort services, in addition to personal care and housekeeping. Family Care is procured at the regional level through a competitive process using a standardized request for proposal (RFP) form. Family Care contractors are monitored through monthly on-site visits by DHS staff. During these visits staff review a stratified sample of both intake and ongoing cases, to determine if the contractor is delivering services according to program standards. If the contractor is not performing satisfactorily, corrective action plans are written. On an annual basis, the contractor's performance is measured against a statewide floor. If the contractor's performance falls below the floor, the contract is not renewed and a new contract is competitively let.

Primary Home Care services include personal care, housekeeping, nurse supervision, and escort services. Primary Home Care contractors are procured through an open enrollment process. Service is monitored through a comprehensive utilization review system that includes site visits to both the contractor's office and the client's home. Each contractor is monitored quarterly. If performance is unsatisfactory, corrective action plans are prepared. A system of provider sanctions is also being developed. These sanctions, which could range from suspension of new referrals to contract cancellation, will be applied to providers identified as poor performers in the utilization review system.

Rate setting for the two programs differs slightly, in recognition of the differences in procurement methodologies. For Family Care, a fixed unit rate is set for each contract, through the competitive process. All agencies responding to a Family Care RFP must bid at or below a statewide ceiling. Unit rates in Family Care ranged from $4.32 an hour to $5.23 an hour in fiscal year 1984, with a statewide average of $4.88, weighted by hours of service in the contracts. For Primary Home Care, a statewide flat rate is used ($5.47 an hour in fiscal year 1984). Both the rate ceiling and flat rate are derived after analysis of annual cost reports submitted by providers.

STEPS IN SYSTEM-BASED CONTRACTING

The Texas Department of Human Services uses a systems approach to procure and arrange home care services. As stated earlier, this comprehensive process goes beyond performance-based contracting in that it considers the entire life of a contracted service, from service definition through contract cancellation. System-based contracting also integrates both service delivery and fiscal expectations early in the design process, thus helping to simplify service administration for both the contractor and the purchasing agency.

The remainder of this chapter contains a detailed description of each of these steps.

Defining Service Requirements

A good service definition is the foundation upon which the rest of the program is built. It is important not to attempt to design the entire program until the following elements have been clearly defined:

- Basic service to be purchased
- Delivery mechanism
- Potential provider base

The definition of these program elements can be shaped by many different considerations. Some of the most significant determinants might include a needs assessment of the target population, input from field staff and consumer groups, existence or need for enabling legislation and regulations, and the experiences of other organizations in delivering similar services.

The service definition selected should be very basic. The intent should be to strip the service down to its core and to build the rest of the program around this basic definition. Some examples of simple and concise definitions of home care services include:

- The delivery of personal care, meal preparation, and housekeeping services in the client's home
- The delivery of a meal to the client's home
- The provision of temporary relief (respite) to the normal caregiver, in the client's home

Once a service definition has been decided, the next area to define is the delivery mechanism—how services will be provided to clients. This stage is often combined with the definition of the provider base. While these two steps may be interrelated, it is important first to look at them separately and then go back and make any necessary adjustments. Some examples of delivery mechanisms are:

- Part-time employees, primarily friends or family members, who only serve one or two clients
- Full-time employees, not family members and friends, who serve a wide variety and number of clients
- Volunteers who are reimbursed only for expenses

The definition of the provider base will specify the type of organization with which the program will be entering into contract to provide the service. Preferably, the definition should assure broad availability of the service, adequate competition, and nonrestraint of trade. In addition, the program may want to identify those potential providers who could be reasonably expected to perform the service and who possess the necessary management skills to meet both fiscal and service expectations. Some potential definitions are:

- A legal entity licensed by the state as a home health agency and certified for reimbursement under Titles XVIII and XIX of the Social Security Act
- Area Agencies on Aging
- Local branches of government or nonprofit agencies

Defining Fiscal Control Expectations

The next major step is to define fiscal expectations. During this step it is necessary to specify the following:

- Unit of service
- Cost reporting mechanism
- Reimbursement methodology
- Auditing process

The unit of service is the smallest common denominator used to designate service delivery for billing and cost analysis. For most attendant care programs a unit of service is one hour of authorized service delivered to the client (see Chapter 3).

After the unit of service is defined, the purchasing agency must spell out its system for reconciling services authorized against services delivered and services billed. Any expectations concerning such items as time sheets, authorization documents, and billing documents must be clearly stated prior to signing a contract, to insure a smooth auditing process.

The next major step is to select a reimbursement methodology. Texas considered three major types: cost reimbursement; cost reimbursement with a unit-rate ceiling; and a flat rate. Based on its judgment of the advantages and disadvantages of each type, Texas chose a flat-rate reimbursement system. This provides predictable costs to the purchaser and predictable cash flow to the contractor. It also focuses negotiation on final costs rather than on each component and allows the contractor to make adjustments in its organization as necessary. This method also simplifies the auditing process; with a flat-rate reimbursement system the audit can primarily focus on reconciling hours authorized with hours delivered and billed.

Texas DHS rejected cost reimbursement as a payment method. The department found that cost reimbursement gave the purchasing agency the least control over costs and the quantity of services purchased. Cost reimbursement with a unit-rate ceiling was viewed as somewhat better because it set an outside limit on costs and at least a minimum expectation for quantity. Both of these methods, however, can require complex and detailed negotiation, monitoring, billing, and auditing for the fiscal portion of the contract. It has been Texas's experience that these methods are not efficient for larger contracts.

Once a program is operating, the purchasing agency needs to collect cost data for monitoring and planning purposes. The contractor's responsibility to provide these data should be clearly spelled out before a contract is signed. Most cost reporting occurs either through the billing process or through periodic cost reports. Under cost reimbursement contracts the contractor is paid based on costs incurred during the service period. Thus, costs are reported as part of the billing process. Where costs are not reported in the billing system, contractors report their costs on an annual or other regular basis. Both methods require an audit in order to assure the quality of the data.

Texas requires its contractors to complete a cost report every 12 months. The cost reports for Family Care and Primary Home Care have the same data elements. This enables the DHS rate-setting staff to compare data by contractor, territory, and program. This helps them determine whether cost variations are caused by internal operations of the specific contractor, by location, or by policy. DHS staff can examine, for example, the cost implications of the Title XIX requirement for registered nurse supervision in Primary Home Care as compared to other levels of supervision in Family Care.

Defining Service Delivery Expectations

Once the basic service has ben defined in operating and fiscal terms, it can be integrated and elaborated by setting service delivery expectations. These expectations are the minimum acceptable requirements for service delivery.

- Each expectation must be measurable. If it cannot be measured, there is no way to know if it happened.
- Each expectation must be discrete. It must have a specific

beginning and end.

- Each expectation must be objective. It should take little, if any, subjective judgment to determine if it occurred.
- Each expectation must be simple. It should be basic enough that a variety of staff can understand it.

In order for the purchasing agency to monitor service expectations on an ongoing basis, it needs to meet standards for performance at critical junctions. For in-home services the standards should address quality, timeliness, accuracy, and continuity. Four examples from among the standards used by DHS are:

- The contract agency must initiate services within 14 days of the date of referral.
- Supervisors must be registered nurses.
- Attendants must not give personal care services until they have shown competence in this area to their supervisor's satisfaction.
- The contract agency must perform services as authorized by the state.

Other expectations are monitored on an exception basis. In general, these include expectations that are costly to monitor, less discrete, or more difficult to quantify. Some examples in Texas include:

- Contract agency employees must not solicit or accept gifts or favors of monetary value from a client or family member as a gift, reward, or payment for services provided to the client.
- The contract agency must not knowingly utilize providers who have symptoms of communicable disease or open infectious wounds.
- The contract agency must fully comply with the Civil Rights Act of 1965 and the Rehabilitation Act of 1973, as amended.

Selecting Providers

Assuming that the provider base defined in the first step includes many potential candidates, providers can be selected by either competitive procurement or provider enrollment. Texas uses both methods: competitive procurement for Family Care and provider enrollment for Primary Home Care. The decision to use competitive procurement in Family Care was made with the intention of getting the most service for the dollar. The provider enrollment in Primary Care complies with federal Health Care Financing Administration requirements intended to insure that clients have freedom of choice.

Texas has considered the use of two basic types of competitive procurement documents: the invitation for bid (IFB) and the request for proposal (RFP). The IFB details the plan of operation that all contractors must follow and sets service delivery and fiscal expectations. The bidder must submit verification that it meets the screening requirements, together with written assurance that it will perform according to the plan of operation and that it will provide service at a certain unit rate. The contract is then awarded to the lowest bidder. The IFB has a very objective selection process. Its weaknesses are that it provides little opportunity to identify innovative approaches and that it offers little chance to screen out weak organizations. Cost becomes the sole criterion for choosing among competing providers.

In the RFP process, the bidder proposes a plan of operation describing how it will meet the expectations and a unit rate at which it will provide the service. Generally, the response also provides information on previous experience. The bidder still must meet the initial screening requirements and assurances. The entire proposal is evaluated and usually the top three or four proposers are invited to negotiate and to amend their proposals before the final evaluation and selection. The RFP process provides the purchaser a better opportunity to evaluate alternative approaches and assess the strengths and weaknesses of bidders. It is, however, a more involved and subjective approach to selection of contractors.

Texas has attempted to combine what it believes to be the best of both methods. The Texas DHS uses an RFP format but only evaluates the proposals of a specified number of lowest bidders. It has found that this process reduces staff time spent on procurement and focuses the staff's efforts on negotiating and evaluating those proposals that are the most competitive. DHS believes this greatly simplifies the selection process yet provides staff with a wider array of selection criteria than the typical IFB process, because proposals are evaluated on the basis of feasibility, quality, and cost.

Obtaining an Agency Plan

The agency plan required of bidders must provide detailed descriptions of their organizational structure, their service delivery plan, and the way they propose to relate to the DHS. For provider enrollment and IFB procurement systems, these descriptions are usually defined solely by the purchaser, in provider manuals and standard contract documents. When services are procured through an RFP, the proposer has more latitude in describing how it proposes to deliver the service.

One of the early RFPs used by Texas allowed the contractor both to bid a rate and to commit to greater service delivery expectations than required in the state's minimum standards. DHS found that this pulled the contractor from two opposite directions, promising higher quality and lower costs. This process caused confusion among bidders as to what aspects of service quality were most important. It also generated difficulties for DHS staff in selecting among proposals that had different strengths and weaknesses and resulted in variations in service quality across the state. Later RFPs did not allow a bidder to commit to stricter standards than the statewide minimums.

Over time, DHS concluded that service quality was primarily dependent upon the contractor's ability to manage a widespread, labor-intensive delivery system. In addition, DHS found that this ability was reflected in the conciseness of the organizational chart, in effective channels of communication, in internal audit and quality control systems, and in the quality of the contractor's payroll system. As a result, Texas revised the RFP it uses for in-home services, to place greater emphasis on program management. Each bidder must now spell out both its agency's internal management structure and a plan of operation that covers the three stages of the contract: start-up, service delivery, and termination.

1. The precontract or start-up phase defines the period before service delivery begins. In this section of the proposal, the bidder states its plan for preparing to take over service operation. These steps may include hiring staff, setting up offices, contracting for home attendants, and building a data base for personnel and payroll.
2. The service delivery stage refers to the bidder's ongoing provision of home care services. In this section of the pro-

posal, the contractor describes internal operations and demonstrates how its service delivery plan will assure that services will be delivered at the level of quality specified by the DHS.

3. The third stage, termination, looks at the eventual point when the bidder will no longer have the contract. In this section the bidder explains how it will cooperate with the state and a new contractor to assure a smooth transition.

In subsequent sections of the proposal, the bidder gives a detailed description of its organization, identifies the entry points for field contract by DHS staff, and specifies the decision-making authority of staff at those points. The bidder is also required to specify the information flow within its organization and state how policy and procedure changes are disseminated throughout its structure. Texas also requires a description of the contractor's internal quality control system, payroll system, and audit trails for services authorized, delivered, and billed.

The last section of the proposal covers the unit-rate bid and a prospective cost report to substantiate the rate. The prospective cost report helps to assure that substantial thought has gone into developing the rate and that the bid is not frivolous.

Monitoring Service Delivery

After the contract is signed and service delivery has begun, DHS's attention focuses on monitoring the ongoing delivery of the service. In some ways this is the most important step in the whole process. Without monitoring and appropriate feedback mechanisms, the impact of planning is lessened. The contractor is informed that its efforts will be monitored and that it will be expected to take the necessary corrective action to remove any deficiencies.

The goal of monitoring is to provide information to contractors and department managers that can be used to identify strengths and weaknesses in the current delivery system. In DHS's view, the monitoring plan must:

- be consistently applied, to insure that all contractors are treated equally
- provide timely feedback, to assure that the contractor has ample time to correct any deficiencies

- be reasonable and not place an inordinate burden on either the contractor or the purchasing agency
- be simple enough not to require constant exception statements or result in misunderstandings between contractors and monitors.

Departmental staff and contractors receive copies of DHS's service control and utilization review monitoring guides. The intent is to let contractors know from the start what is expected and how they will be monitored. DHS reviews records monthly in Family Care and quarterly in Primary Home Care. After a program review is completed, DHS staff and contractors meet together to review the results, in order to reconcile performance with expectations.

Texas has a system for sanctioning Family Care contractors and is developing a system of sanctions for Primary Home Care, to make certain that recommendations for corrective actions are carried out. A well-designed sanctions system must be consistent, reasonable, and enforceable. In particular, its impact on the client, the purchasing agency, and the provider base must be considered. For example, clients may suffer disruption in service while a provider is being sanctioned or suffer from inferior service before a sanction is finally implemented. The purchasing agency has to be willing to spend staff resources on administrative hearings and possibly on court action as well. The provider base could shrink or evaporate if the system is too punitive; also, providers might ignore any attempts to improve services if the system is too cumbersome. Some of the options for sanctions are:

- Corrective action plans
- Suspension of intake
- Vendor hold
- Liquidated damages
- Fines
- Contract cancellation

The main point to remember when developing a monitoring and sanctions system is that the great majority of contractors will do a good job when they understand what is wanted. Monitoring and sanctions systems should not overburden the majority but should quickly and clearly deal with poor performers.

Renewing the Contract Cycle

Once a given contract cycle has been completed, the Texas approach calls for a repeat of the process, starting with the inclusion of any additional service or financial requirements and continuing on to the issuance of a new RFP and contract award.

LINKAGES WITHIN THE SYSTEM

Texas has substantially integrated its service control and fiscal control systems through the statewide use of common-source documents. Essentially, one set of forms is used and built upon to satisfy the majority of information needs. From these source documents, the DHS and its contractors can add and extract information on service plans, authorization dates, time sheets, billing, and statistical performance. This greatly simplifies the auditing process because the necessary paper trail is created in the service delivery process. In addition, with service and fiscal control integrated, certain discrepancies such as those between authorized and actual initiation dates or service levels are substantially eliminated.

Under the Texas system, the integrated process is initiated when a DHS caseworker or nurse authorizes the contractor to provide service. The authorization form includes client identifying information, type and level of service authorized, tasks to be performed, and duration of the authorization. The contractor uses this information to build a detailed task assignment plan and a time sheet, which are then given to the home attendant. The attendant enters, directly onto this form, the hours worked each day in the pay period. The contractor collects the time sheets and uses these and the service authorization form to prepare the billing document. To help in this regard, the DHS sends the contractor a preprinted billing form; usually all the contractor has to do is enter the number of hours delivered per client and the dollars billed per client and then compute the total number of billed hours and dollars.

Service control personnel review these standardized forms to determine compliance for service initiation dates, service breaks, and service authorization. These forms also provide the information needed to review supervisory visits, attendant competency, and other performance expectations. The auditing process then uses these forms plus billing documents to reconcile hours authorized versus hours delivered and hours billed. Since the fiscal control and service control processes are mirror images, a contractor with a good service contract record should have a clean audit. In addition, by issuing the same source documents for performance measurements, billing, and auditing, costly paperwork duplication is substantially reduced.

POTENTIAL FOR REPLICATION

Texas's conceptual approach to contracting can be used by any purchasing organization. It assumes (1) that the organization is interested not only in the design and implementation of services but also in their ongoing efficient management, and (2) that there is a willingness to question current operational practices. Essentially it involves reviewing services using a systems approach, and building a contract process that will meet the service and fiscal management needs of the purchasing agency.

A key to the successful implementation of Texas's system-based contracting was involving all those with an interest in service and fiscal management of home care in the development of the contracting system. This process was one of building consensus for the change. Although time-consuming, the process meant that the end product was supported throughout the organization. The organizational entities involved in the review encompassed both the vertical and horizontal structures of the home care service system. This helped assure that the management requirements of the delivery system, from the client on up to the executive staff, were met and that the management requirements of the various support groups in the organization, such as data systems, fiscal audit, and legal, would also be satisfied. Broadening the vested interest in the product in this way built consensus on the contracting system and thereby helped assure the project's success.

While some of the practices Texas uses in its contracted program were designed for large delivery systems and demand technical sophistication, others do not. For instance, unit-rate contracting requires providers with good cash flow management skills. Texas's rate-setting methodology makes use of microcomputers to build rates, using both detailed cost reports and economic models.

While home care programs may not be readily able to adopt unit-rate contracting or Texas's rate-setting methods, other of Texas's practices could be easily adapted by other programs. Texas's performance standards, monitoring guides, and RFP documents all could be helpful to other programs involved in redesigning the contracting process or reviewing their programs.

9

Unit-Rate Contracting in the State of Washington

The Department of Social and Health Services (DSHS) in the State of Washington has established the practice of purchasing chore services through fixed-price, unit-rate contracts. Its use of unit-rate contracts is linked to the emphasis that such contracts place on service delivery. In addition, fixed prices make reimbursement administratively easier than is the case with line-item cost reimbursement.

PROGRAM BACKGROUND

Washington's chore services program is designed to prevent unnecessary residential care placement by providing a range of household and personal care services to elderly and disabled adults (including those who are developmentally disabled). Chore services are delivered through two programs: the contracted program and the individual provider program. What distinguishes the two is the tasks performed. Personal care, requiring specialized training, and attendant care are provided through the individual provider program. General personal care and household tasks are provided through the contracted program. It is the contracted program that is the subject of this chapter, since that is where the practice of unit-rate contracting has been applied. (In the individual provider program, the client employs the worker.)

In December 1985, 10,815 clients were provided with chore services, 8,254 of whom were served through the contracted program. About three-quarters of the clients were over 60 years old. Funding for chore services in the state's 1985–1987 biennial budget was $57 million. Approximately 51 percent of this amount came from the Social Services Block Grant, and 49 percent came from the state's general fund.

Client eligibility is governed by state legislation. The law mandates that both financial eligibility and service eligibility be assessed before chore services can be authorized.

A standardized client review questionnaire is used to determine both the degree and level of service need and to provide consistency in the authorization of chore service hours. For each task allowed under the program the assessment determines (1) if any assistance is needed, (2) if assistance is or can be provided by sources other than the core services program, and (3) the degree of assistance needed from the program. A score is assigned to each task and a chart translates the total score into the maximum number of hours that can be authorized. In fiscal 1985, clients received an average of 20 hours of chore services a month.

Services are provided at no charge to adults aged 18 and over who are recipients of Supplemental Security Income, SSI State Supplementation, the state-limited casualty program of medical care, or have gross income below 30 percent of the state median income. (This would mean a gross income of less than $396 per month for a single person or $518 per month for a couple.) The state legislature mandated that the DSHS develop a sliding scale of participation for those clients with income above 30 percent of the state median income (SMI). Clients with incomes between 30 and 50 percent of SMI are reduced one hour from the service authorization for each 1 percent of income over 30 percent of SMI. Clients with incomes over 50 percent of SMI are reduced an additional two hours from the service authorization for each percent of income over 50 percent of SMI. (Fifty percent of SMI is equal to $660 per month for a single person or $863 per month for a couple.)

The law also requires that resources cannot exceed $10,000 for one person and $15,000 for a couple. These resource limitations are similar to the State Senior Citizens Services Act that provides funds for services for older persons.

The overall administration and development of the chore service program is the responsibility of the Bureau of Aging and Adult Services in the DSHS. Eligibility determination is delegated to case workers in the department's Community Service offices around the state. The responsibility of providing a system for delivering chore services to eligible clients is contracted by the bureau to 10 Area Agency of Aging offices. Under the terms of this contract, AAA's are required to enter into subcontracts for the provision of chore services.

Contracts between the AAA's and providers must conform to state policies and procedures and to program standards specified in the contract between the Bureau of Aging and Adult Services and each Area Agency on Aging. Among these is the policy that contracts be on a unit-rate basis and that the process for awarding contracts be a competitive one using requests for proposals (RFP's).

Competition for chore services is required by the bureau as a cost containment measure intended to lower or at least stabilize the unit rate. But another, more direct cost containment measure is part of the rate-setting process: a legislated cap on the unit rate for chore services. The cap was imposed as a budget control measure.

The number of potential service providers has greatly increased since the chore services program was contracted out. As a result, there is competition for the chore services contracts in all areas in the state. This has helped to keep rates down. There are currently 18 chore services providers in Washington State. Two of the providers are public agencies, and the balance are private nonprofit agencies.

At the beginning of Washington's program in 1979, AAA's were allowed to set their own rates. This resulted in diversity in the range of hourly rates across the state. But from the imposition of a cap on the hourly rate in 1981 (which has been adjusted only by a percentage increase for inflation) to 1986, most of the hourly rates reached the allowable maximum of $6.16.

IMPLEMENTATION OF UNIT-RATE CONTRACTING

Washington has used unit-rate contracts to buy chore services since 1979, when it first established its contracted program. Prior to this, chore services were provided only by individual workers, whom it was up to the client to recruit and employ. The state was dissatisfied with the practice of making clients responsible for the employment of service workers because it was feared that the same disabling conditions that brought them to the program in the first place could hamper their ability to carry out these responsibilities. The goal in moving to a system where the state would purchase the chore services was to assure services to clients who might be unable to recruit their own workers.

Two demonstration projects and some other experiences under the state's Senior Citizens Services Act had given the state experience with unit-rate contracting. This feature of unit-rate contracts complemented the state's desire to assure a high quality of service delivery and led to the decision to adopt this form of contracting in the chore services program.

Distinctive Features

What is distinctive about the unit-rate method of contracting is the fact that what is being purchased and the purchase price are both defined in terms of a common unit of measure: an hour of chore services. Typically, an AAA contracts with a chore service organization to buy up to a certain number of hours of chore services at a fixed price for each hour delivered. The method therefore directly ties contract payments to the hours of service delivered. This is in sharp contrast to the case where expenditures are incurred against a line-item budget and there is no guaranteed connection between expense and service level.

A unit-rate contract may ultimately purchase the same number of service hours as a conventional line-item contract for the same dollar amount, but payment under the two contracts and therefore fiscal accountability are quite different. Under the unit-rate method, payment is tied to an accounting of the number of authorized hours of chore services that have been delivered, and the provider is paid the agreed unit price for each hour of service delivered. Under the line-item method, payment is normally tied to an accounting of the allowable costs and expenditures incurred against the line items in the contract budget. While line-item contracts also involve accounting for the hours of service delivered, this is only for reporting purposes and not for cost validation and payment purposes.

Unit-rate contracts simplify the billing and payments process. By tying the service units to the unit price, validation for the bills by the AAA's is a matter of reconciling billed and authorized service hours. This eliminates the additional process of reconciling billed costs against the line-item budget. In Washington this has speeded up the invoicing and reimbursement process for AAA's and has freed more of their time for program development and technical assistance.

Control over Provider Performance

Some home care administrators fear that the separation of payment from the line-item budget will lead to loss of control over provider agencies. Washington has not found that to be the case. Washington's incorporation of performance standards in the contracts provides control over provider performance. The RFP process used to award contracts requires the providers to submit technical and management information as well as price proposals. These must specify in detail what they will provide, how they will do it, and at what price. These technical and management proposals specify the operational policies and procedures for which the provider can be held accountable. Moreover, the price proposal must be based on a line-item budget, enabling the AAA and the state to negotiate cost elements as part of the process of negotiating the unit price. Providers are also required to submit periodic cost reports throughout the contract period, with information on actual costs measured against the same line-item budget as in the price proposal. It is on the basis of these cost data that the state and AAA are able to build a cost history and evaluate whether the unit rate being paid is the fair one. If it is found not to be fair, the data provide the basis for setting a new rate at the time the contract is up for renegotiation. Alternatively, there may be a provision built into the contract that allows the rate to be renegotiated within the contract period, under certain circumstances.

In Washington's experience, giving up direct control over line items has not meant loss of control over providers. What it has meant is that, once the AAA's and the providers have adjusted to the new system, they can develop a relationship that centers on the content of the service being provided. As stated by one spokesperson for an area agency, "Detailed analysis of line items does not change the amount of service delivered."

Seven Key Tasks

As implemented in Washington, the practice of fixed unit-rate contracting involves a process with seven key tasks:

1. Establishing a common definition of the service to be provided
2. Describing a standard service unit at its most discrete level (for example, one hour, one visit, one meal)
3. Writing standards for the delivery of the service
4. Developing an RFP for use in soliciting bids from service providers (competitive procurement)
5. Scoring the RFP submission on objective criteria and selecting a provider
6. Negotiating and writing a clear and concise contract
7. Judging provider performance and accountability

An eighth task that has operated in practice in Washington is the statewide cap on the chore services rate as a further cost containment measure. This need not be done to put the unit-rate concept into practice, however.

Responsibility for the seven tasks is shared at the state and local level. At the outset the Bureau of Aging and Adult Services was responsible for defining the service unit, tasks, and standards for the program; subsequently, definitions of tasks and standards have been revised on the basis of AAA and contractor input. The state designed the original format for the RFP and set standards for the review of proposals. From information provided by AAA's on the number of current clients, the state projected caseload growth over the biennial budget and the state was able to set an hourly cap that would not exceed its budget. Final negotiated rates have always been approved by the state, although this has become *pro forma*, given the cap on rates.

Definitions and Standards of Service

Currently, the bureau is still responsible for developing the definitions and standards for the program. It sets the maximum statewide rate and performs or contracts for statewide evaluation of chore services. AAA's are responsible for issuing RFP's, establishing the proposal review procedure, writing contracts, monitoring service providers for contract compliance and client satisfaction, conducting audits, and reimbursing providers for service units delivered.

Definitions of service and standards are central to the Washington approach. Before a unit of service is chosen on which payment can be made, the service must be adequately defined. The definition should lead logically to assigning the unit on the basis of time (hour), task (visit), or product (meal). The unit must also be described as discretely as possible in relation to the service definition.

The next step—or perhaps an intermediary step—in describing the unit is writing standards for service delivery. How "thin" or "rich" the service will be depends on these standards. In turn, the standards determine how costly the unit will be to purchase. Implementing these may mean that other costs must be added to the basic unit rate. For example, consider a meals program where the unit is one meal. The cost of that meal will vary depending on whether the standards specify it is to be cold or hot. If standards further specify it is to meet one-third of the recommended dietary allowance for one day, portion sizes may increase, food costs may rise, and the rate may have to go up. For chore services, the rate is directly affected by "add-ons" to the basic rate of pay for one hour of chore service. In Washington in 1985, wages and benefits for a chore worker typically came to $4.50 an hour. To this would be added $1.20 an hour for indirect costs (administrative salaries and office overhead). Another $0.15 an hour would be added as profit, or excess reimbursement for nonprofits; and there are transportation costs for workers, which may come to $0.30 an hour; and so on. As more things are added on, the rate goes up.

Proposal and Contract

The RFP sets the stage for everything that happens after a contractor is selected. If something is not anticipated in the RFP, it is very difficult to rectify later. This is especially true if the contract is to be for a fixed unit price. The RFP must include the service definition, unit, and standards. It must include the anticipated number of units to be purchased. It must specify administrative requirements. In short, it must include anything that impacts cost. Finally, it must include the forms and procedures for documenting and reporting service delivery and costs.

In Washington, cost is not the sole factor in determining whether or not an agency receives a contract. Management capability and technical expertise are also scored; in fact, their combined scoring outweighs cost as a factor, so an agency may receive a contract even though its unit cost is higher than another. Therefore, competitive bidding alone does not necessarily contain costs.

A clear, concise contract must be negotiated which sets the unit rate to be paid, the number of units to be provided, how and where the service is to be provided, and what reports are to be generated. Some negotiation on cost and operating procedures may occur between the AAA and the selected chore provider.

Cost Report

Once a project is under way, the most important report the Area Agency on Aging receives from the chore contractor is the cost report. This may be collected quarterly, semiannually, or annually. Washington believes that it is essential to collect more data than simple information on how a provider expends funds received under the contract. The report should gather all costs associated with delivering the service, including complete revenue and cost data covering donations and client fees, profit, unspent funds, and the cost of equipment amortization. The actual number of service units provided during the cost reporting period is then divided into the total actual cost to determine unit cost. This is the only way that the provider and an AAA know if the rate being paid is more or less than the actual cost of providing one unit of service.

Since contracting for chore services is primarily an AAA responsibility, the cost of administering Washington's contracting must be included in the state's contracts with its AAA's. Nine of the AAA's receive $76,772 per two-year contract period for chore services administration; the other AAA, the largest in the state, receives $148,064. The bureau itself has one chore services program manager, and other bureau staff provide assistance in contract development, accounting, reporting, budget projections, evaluation, and technical assistance.

Audits

In auditing a fixed-price unit-rate contract, the purpose is not to check on the allowability of expenditures, as is the case in a cost reimbursement contract.[1] The purpose is instead to confirm the integrity and accuracy of the financial statement (including cost reports) and to account for the provision of units. This involves checking that all costs are reported, verifying the soundness of the accounting system, and verifying service delivery. AAA's are required to audit their contractors at least every two years.

Performance Measurement

Monitoring, or performance measurement, should include both fiscal and program monitoring. In Washington, quarterly cost reports are received by AAA's from providers. The reports provide a total cost picture (including all revenues) for the provision of the service. This makes it possible to judge the fairness and reasonableness of the price being paid and also provides a basis for negotiating a new fixed price if circumstances warrant. AAA's usually verify service delivery by spot-sampling client records against worker time sheets. The AAA must ascertain that the hours provided to each client did not exceed the allocated hours (units) for that client. AAA's also review monthly program reports and monitor the contractor annually for compliance with contract provisions, including the managerial and technical plans incorporated in the original proposal.

PROGRAM IMPACT

The greatest impact of fixed-price unit-rate contracting has been on provider agencies. On the negative side, unit rates can work against small agencies, creating cash flow problems that make it hard for them to cover start-up costs and monthly payrolls and make them more sensitive to changes in the monthly volume of units. Over time, AAA's have worked with the smaller agencies in developing some solutions to their difficulties. For example, Sea-Mar, one of the chore services contractors in King County,

---

[1]Federal regulations [45 Code of Federal Regulations (CFR) Part 74] provide an explanation of the federal rules governing unit-rate contracting.

was initially forced to take out short-term bank loans to meet its payroll. In conjunction with the AAA, they worked out a plan where a variable unit rate was paid for services delivered. In the first three months a higher unit rate was paid, to provide better cash flow. This rate was reduced during the rest of the contract year, bringing it into line with the average rate specified in the contract. Other solutions to providers' problems have included the following:

- Where capital acquisitions were a problem, separate line-item cost reimbursements have been used. The separate contract makes it possible for the provider to recover costs in one lump sum rather than amortizing the cost over the contract period.
- Because the State of Washington does not allow advances to service providers, to assist with cash flow difficulties some AAA's reimburse contractors twice a month. The first warrant is based on 85 percent of the previous month's expenditures. The second warrant equals the difference between actual monthly expenditures and the first warrant.

While the introduction of unit-rate contracts has produced difficulties for some providers, it has also benefited providers by giving them budget flexibility. Under many line-item contracts, amendments must be made each time expenditures change for a particular line item. Under a unit-rate contract, provider agencies can alter cost centers within budgets without AAA permission. While accounting requirements have not changed, reimbursement has been speeded up. Providers no longer have to prepare line-item documentation to verify billing requests, nor do AAA's have to check these prior to payment. On average, Washington's AAA's can pay bills within a two-week period.

Detailed budget information must still be kept. As noted above, a line-item budget is used to negotiate the rate. While this budget may be deviated from by the provider, cost reports are completed using the same budget line items, thus enabling comparison of actual cost experience with the proposed budget.

A benefit to Washington State of the fixed-price unit-rate contract is that it does away with the cost settlement process and gives providers an incentive to be efficient. This benefit may also have a cost, as the state cannot recover any amount of surplus over expenditure generated by providers who can deliver the service for less than the unit rate. Washington has reviewed this cost to its program. In 1985, based on cost reports, 11 providers experienced a profit ranging from $0.03 to $0.28 an hour, 4 providers had a loss ranging from $0.11 to $0.60 an hour, and 2 providers broke even. Statewide, the rate paid exceeded the unit cost by $0.02 an hour. This resulted in $180,302 in overexpenditures, or a profit that represented 1 percent of the chore budget. This cost the state and the AAA's less, in their view, than it would have cost to go through a cost settlement process.

As far as clients are concerned, the major impact of the new chore service program has been the decision to contract the service out rather than pay the client directly. In the former payment scheme, the clients had to employ their own workers. In the contracted program the worker is employed by the provider agency and assigned to the client. The client, therefore, does not have to deal with the inconvenience and paperwork or worry about the legal obligations of being an employer. The introduction of unit-rate contracting in particular did not alter in any way the benefits of the broader decision to contract out the program.

The changes that unit-rate contracting sets in motion in relation to financial management tasks might be characterized as not major in relation to budgeting, accounting, auditing, and performance measurement. The most significant change is in the payment system, which is on the basis of units of service rather than expenditures. Budgeting and accounting processes see little change, with perhaps two exceptions. AAA's are in a proactive position of specifying what services they want and how much of them they want to buy from providers, whereas under line-item contracts this tends to be a matter of what the provider says it can provide. Second, unit-cost data facilitate projecting caseloads and budgets more accurately. This is true for the AAA or the state, depending on which level has the responsibility.

POTENTIAL FOR REPLICATION

To implement the unit-rate practice successfully elsewhere, there must be strong backing from the state agency. This backing must be given with the full knowledge that traditional controls such as line-item budgets will not be in place. It also must be supported by having available the technical expertise needed to implement, monitor, and troubleshoot the process.

The types of resistance that might be encountered include fear on the part of AAA's and the state of unreasonable provider profits or overpayments, fear that a sufficient volume of service to break even cannot be attained, a perception that the concept will be difficult to master, fear on the part of the provider that reimbursement will not cover costs, and providers' concern about their ability to write a competitive proposal.

In dealing with these and other possible problems, the following actions can be taken: The state and AAA's should identify service units before unit rates are negotiated; AAA's should be thoroughly educated in unit-rate methods of contracting, monitoring, auditing, and reimbursing; and provider agencies should be eased into the unit-rate system by permitting them to use variable rates or cost reimbursement for a while before switching them over to fixed rates.

There are cases where unit-rate contracting could be the wrong approach. It may not be appropriate in small agencies with cash flow problems, in a brand-new service, in services where provision levels fluctuate greatly from month to month, or in cases where the unit of service cannot be defined discretely.

For the system to be implemented successfully, the AAA's must be fairly well trained in fiscal and accounting procedures and must be skilled at negotiating with provider agencies. Also, it is important that both state and local levels agree on the principles of unit-rate contracting. Finally, while it is difficult to say with certainty whether Washington's experience would have been different in the absence of the legislative cap on rates, the state staff believe that the unit-rate approach could have worked as well without the stimulus of the cap.

10

Two-Tiered Contracting in New York City

In 1980, New York City's Office of Home Care Services implemented a two-tiered reimbursement system for its contracts with agencies that provide Medicaid-funded personal care services. This system was put in place when a large caseload that previously had been handled by independent providers (individual home attendants hired by the client) was transferred to the care of nonprofit vendor agencies. The first tier of payment was established to cover direct-service costs, home attendant wages, and fringe benefits. The second tier of payment was designed to cover administrative costs. The practice enabled New York City to maintain better control over administrative costs while providing advance funding for service costs to small nonprofit providers who lack start-up capital. This approach to contracting offers an interesting contrast to that of the State of Washington, described in the previous chapter.

PROGRAM BACKGROUND

New York City's Home Attendant Program is administered by

the Human Resources Administration (HRA), a municipal agency that is responsible for providing a very broad range of social service and income assistance programs. The program operates in the five counties (boroughs) that make up the City of New York. Under New York State law, the city is treated as a single social service district (elsewhere in the state, districts are single counties).

The objective of the New York program is to help clients remain in their own homes and to prevent institutionalization. In light of the severe shortage of nursing home beds in the city, which is due to a very high level of demand for service, sustaining elderly persons in their own homes has been given very high priority by the city administration.

The program of personal care services is entirely financed under Medicaid. Its budget of $448 million for fiscal year 1986 made it the largest Medicaid personal care program in the country. It served in 1986 over 30,000 clients, most of whom were elderly women who live alone.

Eligibility for home attendant services as required under Medicaid is tied both to financial eligibility for medical assistance and to medical need. Because the city and state have elected to include the medically needy in the eligible population, in addition to the categorically eligible, the eligibility pool is significantly larger than it is in states that have not opted to include the medically needy in their service population.

The application process for home attendant services is initiated by the client or a representative of the client contacting one of HRA's community-based field offices, either in person, by telephone, or by mail. A physician's statement documenting medical need is required from each potential beneficiary. Once the physician's statement is received, an HRA case manager visits the prospective client and conducts a social assessment. The case manager determines the appropriateness of home care, explores possibilities for the participation of relatives and neighbors in the plan of care, and recommends a service plan.

The case manager's report and the physician's statement are submitted to a team of physicians, nurses, and medical social workers at HRA's Office of Home Care Services. This central team reviews the medical and social factors in each case and authorizes the type and level of care. Home visits by the central staff are made only in selected cases where there is a question concerning the extent or precise nature of a beneficiary's needs.

After HRA has authorized service and certified Medicaid eligibility, the Office of Home Care Services assigns the case to a nonprofit vendor agency under contract with the city. Prior to 1980, HRA relied solely on independent contractors for these services, but the agency is now committed to providing all services through community-based nonprofit vendor agencies.

HRA maintains responsibility for follow-up, case management, and periodic reevaluations. Telephone contacts and home visits are part of this ongoing process. Case managers work with service providers to resolve any problems or complaints that beneficiaries may have. HRA contracts with five certified home health agencies for the Medicaid-required nursing assessment and supervision of personal care clients.

Home attendants assist clients with cleaning, shopping, meal preparation, bathing, grooming, toileting, and ambulating. Clients receive from 6 to 168 service hours per week, depending on their functional limitations and on the availability of family or neighbors to assist with their care. Unlike Texas's Medicaid-financed personal care program or Washington's fixed-price home care program, discussed elsewhere in this book, New York City's Home Attendant Program does not have any maximum client service limits. Thus, its average number of client service hours is higher than in those programs. In 1985, the average came to about 50 home attendant hours per client per week.

Vendors under contract with HRA to provide home attendant services are selected competitively. Requests for proposals (RFPs) are issued for a particular geographic area in the city in which vendors are being sought. The areas used for this purpose generally encompass at least two of the city's 59 community districts. Community districts each encompass a population of between 100,000 and 250,000 residents. Currently, some 64 providers are under contract with HRA's Home Attendant Program.

IMPLEMENTATION OF TWO-TIERED CONTRACTING

Rationale

The Office of Home Care Services established the two-tiered contract system in 1980 when it switched from the practice of using individuals hired by the client as home attendants to that of contracting with nonprofit agencies for the provision of personal care services. The two-tiered contract adopted by New York City can by and large be viewed as a tool that was designed to accommodate a variety of different fiscal issues related to developing and contracting with a network of provider agencies.

The decision to move from individual providers stemmed from several problems associated with that practice. One concern was that the federal government might require the city to take on employer's responsibilities for Social Security, tax withholding, and other benefit programs. Another concern was that the individual providers were often not trained and there was only limited monitoring of their work. Furthermore, the program was growing rapidly and HRA's administrative resources were having difficulty keeping pace with a growing administrative workload, especially in obtaining adequate back-up data to support biweekly paychecks for thousands of attendants. The result was that home attendants often experienced problems in getting paid for their services in a timely manner. There was concern that this problem created a potential for service disruption by attendants who are often their clients' lifelines.

As a result of these problems, HRA saw the need for a new service delivery mechanism that would settle the issues of responsibility for employee benefit deductions as well as for attendant training and supervision, and that would assure that attendants received regular paychecks. It was decided that the best method of accomplishing these objectives was to contract with vendors to employ the attendants and oversee the delivery of services. Following that decision, HRA had to address what it wanted its contract system to look like, what fiscal controls it wanted, and how it was going to put the system in place. The two-tiered approach emerged from the series of policy choices made in response to these questions.

Reliance on nonprofits seemed a logical choice. In New York City nearly 70 percent of all social services and about half of all government-financed health expenditures are provided by nonprofit agencies. The city's nonprofit sector includes both large, established voluntary bodies who operate citywide and smaller organizations that operate only in their local communities and whose boards, staff, and clients reflect the cultural and racial diversity of the city's neighborhoods. In considering how the Home Attendant Program could best respond to the diverse client population, HRA felt that organizations based in local communities could more easily locate home attendants who could establish positive relationships with clients, because they speak the client's language or prepare food in a familiar way, or for other comparable reasons. Moreover, for a decentralized service being delivered in the client's home, neighborhood-based organizations were felt to be better positioned to monitor the quality of care being delivered than an agency operating from elsewhere in the city. Taken together, these factors led HRA to decide that its home care program should be operated largely at the community level and that, insofar as feasible, the vendors should be nonprofit organizations based in the communities they were serving.

Developing the System

The commitment to a decentralized, community-based provider system meant that a large number of providers would be required. While there were some experienced agencies in the potential provider base, a good portion of the provider supply had to come from community-based groups that were not experienced in running programs that employed large numbers of people and involved substantial fiscal management responsibilities. The nature of the provider base on which the city was going to rely, plus the more general concern of containing costs in what was already a sizable program, led HRA to decide that it wanted tight fiscal controls in the contract system. For this and other reasons, contracting on a unit-rate basis was rejected at that time. HRA decided to utilize a strictly cost-based reimbursement approach.

The next step in developing the contract program was to establish a cost framework for the contracts. Lacking historical cost data, HRA had to find another means of developing parameters for contract costs. The direct-service cost elements were not difficult to project, since the wages paid to home attendants under the individual provider program were known and the package of benefits could be calculated. What was more difficult was projecting administrative costs. HRA set out to develop budgets reflecting what it considered reasonable administrative costs. Because vendors are required to screen, hire, train, supervise, and pay attendants regardless of how many hours they might work, HRA perceived administrative costs more as a function of the size of caseload than of the number of service hours being delivered. It therefore wanted to assure that agencies serving comparable numbers of clients would receive comparable administrative payments. To guide the provider in developing contract proposals, HRA produced a series of model budgets for agencies handling different sizes of caseloads. These became part of the RFP and guided negotiation of contract budgets.

Providers were selected from the respondents to the city-issued RFP. Some of the selected contractors were members of the city's established social services community, but many others were small groups with strong community ties. These small groups generally had little experience with fiscal management and had no capital to cover start-up costs or lags in reimbursements. As a result, HRA's financial management system had to address these constraints in order to get a large enough supply of providers. Specifically, if the goal of guaranteeing uninterrupted service delivery under the new system was not to be jeopardized, HRA had to design a fiscal management system that could accommodate the cash flow needs of new programs and small community-based agencies. These new entities, many of them separate from any established sponsoring group, lacked resources to cover biweekly payrolls of $65,000 to $120,000 until they received HRA's payment for services rendered. Unless this problem could be resolved, the new delivery mechanism, like the old one, might not guarantee payroll and therefore might threaten continuity of care for the client.

To accommodate the needs of the vendor agencies, HRA's home care administrators and analysts developed a reimbursement system split into two tiers that separated home attendant payroll from vendor administrative costs. This system enabled HRA to advance payroll funds to community-based agencies and still retain strict control over administrative costs.

Under HRA's system, the first tier was established to pay vendors in advance for direct-service costs, providing biweekly payments for home attendant wages and fringe benefits on an advance basis throughout the program year. Home attendants received $3.35 to $4.25 per hour in wages, depending on their seniority and union affiliation. HRA mandated that vendor agencies provide their home attendants with a package of fringe benefits that included 10 days of sick leave, 10 days of annual leave, paid leave to attend training, Social Security, and Unemployment Insurance. In addition, HRA provided health insurance and disability coverage. The total package was valued at about $6.00 per hour. A vendor's advance payment, referred to as an authorized service payment, was calculated by HRA based on a fixed percentage of the agency's authorized service hours for a two-week period. The advance payments were generated not by any vendor request but by HRA.

HRA maintained an automated client file which contained each client's authorization period, allowable weekly service hours, and designated provider. Every two weeks, HRA used this file to generate a "claims forecast" showing the total service hours each vendor was authorized to provide. HRA then used this forecast to calculate each vendor's Tier I Authorized Service Payment (ASP). By tying the ASP to the active client file, the city felt it would have a solid basis for estimating the amount of money necessary to assure vendors' ability to meet payroll.

The vendors' responsibility in relation to the Tier I expenditures was the same as under any other contract. It submitted a bill to HRA for the services that had been delivered, based on payroll tapes that were generated from home attendant time sheets. These bills had to survive an edit against HRA files. In order to be accepted as valid they were checked for client service authorization limits, eligibility, and vendor certification. Only valid bills could be submitted by the city to the state and federal governments for Medicaid reimbursement. If, at year's end, a vendor's advances exceeded billable services provided, the surplus was recouped and used to offset the advance.

The second tier covered vendor administrative costs. Before a prospective vendor signed a contract with HRA, contract managers and vendor representatives negotiated a line-item administrative budget covering staff salaries and fringe benefits, rent, utilities, supplies, and equipment. Model administrative budgets developed by HRA specifically for the home attendant program formed the basis for these negotiations.

Under Tier II, HRA provided a limited advance at the outset of the contract period to cover administrative costs. In order to replenish administrative funds, vendors submitted monthly line-item statements to their HRA contract manager, detailing the prior month's expenditures and forecasting current cash needs. These statements were then reviewed to ensure that vendors were spending at a rate consistent with their annual line-item allocation and that the funds were needed to meet expenses coming due within the next month. Successful completion of this review triggered a payment to the vendor. Again, the auditing cost settlement mechanism was used to recoup any funds paid in excess of actual allowable expenditures.

PROGRAM IMPACT

In its first years of operation, the two-tiered reimbursement system and the move to a contracted program served HRA's primary goals well. While the Home Attendant Program grew from a payroll of $236 million and a caseload of 20,600 clients in 1981 to a payroll of $448 million and a caseload of over 30,000 clients in 1986, the vendor system enabled HRA to cope with this expansion and strengthen its service. Payless paydays are no longer a problem for attendants. The administrative resources of the vendors have improved the program's capacity to provide continuous care, more frequent nursing supervision of clients, and more nursing supervision and training of the attendants.

The primary contribution of the two-tiered reimbursement system to this has been that it has enabled HRA to develop and nurture new home care service organizations by addressing their problems of start-up costs and cash flow. With the system in place, HRA has found no lack of competition for home attendant contracts: Having started out with 37 contracts, HRA at present has contracts with over 60 agencies. Most vendors begin with a contract for 200 or 400 cases, serving clients within their own community district and perhaps an adjoining district. Vendors that exhibit strong fiscal and programmatic performance are often awarded expansion in caseload capacity as well as service area. At this point, most community districts receive service from more than one vendor.

In addition, the two-tiered system has permitted HRA to meet its goal of strict cost-based reimbursement. The line-item administrative budget has enabled HRA to exercise close control over its contractors' administrative spending. The Home Attendant Program has neither experienced problems with misuse of funds nor with vendors accumulating large surpluses because of the inherent difficulty in matching a unit rate to actual expenditures.

These important benefits do, however, carry substantial administrative costs. To enable the system to operate smoothly, contract managers must invest substantial time in assisting vendors in setting up fiscal systems that can accommodate the client-specific information requirements of Medicaid billing. Contract managers must monitor fiscal performance and offer technical assistance while at the same time measuring performance against other program objectives such as compliance with state regulatory requirements. Because the Home Attendant Program serves an expanding clientele, contract managers are squeezed between providing start-up assistance to new providers and working with existing agencies to correct problems they have encountered. Contract managers, many of whom come from service rather than fiscal backgrounds, have difficulty balancing these demands.

The reimbursement system also complicates HRA's efforts to forecast future needs. Because vendors receive advances from which HRA may later recoup funds based on a year-end audit, actual program expenditures are not known until after the cost settlement process is complete. Vendors do not always agree with the audit findings, and HRA has found itself reviewing audits and arbitrating among competing claims.

Finally, by paying vendors in advance, HRA has bestowed an unintended benefit on the State of New York because it has paid 100% of the service cost up front and only later billed the state for the approximately 75% of these costs that are paid for by state and federal contributions. In contrast, other Medicaid services are paid through the state's Medicaid Management Information System (MMIS), with the state covering the full cost as billed and then seeking the city's contribution later. MMIS has not made advance payments like those made to home attendant vendors. Because city dollars have funded the vendors' advance service payments, the city has risked taking a financial loss if vendors spend the funds but never submit enough valid bills to enable the city to claim state and federal reimbursement for these expenditures.

Under a mandate from the State of New York, HRA began preparing in 1986 to convert the system to the MMIS. Using the data generated during the existence of the two-tiered advance payment system, a series of unit rates were to be derived. Home attendant agencies, now well established, under MMIS would bill the state directly for home attendant hours, after editing their bills against HRA's prior approval records. HRA has approached this conversion with confidence that the vendors are firmly established and their fiscal management capabilities are well developed. The extra level of support that the two-tiered system provided, which once was required to nurture their programs, had become unnecessary.

LINKAGES TO FISCAL MANAGEMENT

As prior discussion has indicated, the auditing function is the key to reconciling providers' bills for service with the advance service payments as well as reconciling billed administrative costs with actual administrative costs. Following HRA uniform audit guidelines, a city-designated independent certified public accountant audits each vendor agency every six months. These audits review compliance with key contract provisions as well as the agencies' financial records. While the accounting systems required to support the two-tiered contracts are not different from those for other forms of contracts, the audits require reconciling two sets of payment records, one for each tier, instead of a single payment record.

An important drawback of the two-tiered advance reimbursement system is the difficulty in linking it to budgeting and performance measurement. Determining total service cost and vendor accountability for funds advanced must await completion of the annual audit, often several months after the fiscal year's end and well after budget forecasts are completed. To overcome this difficulty, contract managers have developed interim measures of vendor accountability so that annual funding decisions can be based on vendor performance in several areas such as progress in correcting cited audit exceptions from prior years or compliance with state regulations concerning provider monitoring and training. Vendors with the lowest rankings are placed on probation and assisted through corrective action plans. The rare vendor that does not display sufficient progress is not offered a new contract when the term expires.

POTENTIAL FOR REPLICATION

The Office of Home Care Services' two-tiered reimbursement system provides a useful basis for moving from use of individual attendants to contracted service delivery. It is an approach to contracting that served New York City well when it had no information on how contracted provision was going to work. It allowed for exercising control over provider agencies and nurturing expansion of the provider market. As summed up by one HRA staff member, the two-tiered system offered new nonprofit vendors "a bicycle with training wheels."

The system is primarily suited to governments that want to contract for service delivery and want to encourage community-based organizations without their own capital resources to become providers. There would appear to be little advantage in using the system where the provider base is established or has the capacity to cover start-up costs and fluctuations in cash flow.

For those who might want to replicate the two-tiered system, an obvious precondition is having the authority to advance contract funds. A second precondition is having sufficient administrative resources to provide the vendors the technical assistance necessary to develop and implement sound fiscal management and control systems. HRA's experience would also suggest that from the start the system should be planned and introduced to providers as a mechanism for getting the program under way in the short term. Those replicating the system need to plan, as HRA did, for gradually moving established vendors to a modified "paid-as-billed" system—which provides limited advances at the outset of the program year followed by further payments only upon submission of paid bills—and eventually to a payment system based on a unit rate.

A major selling point of the two-tiered system is its capacity to stimulate the development of small community-based provider agencies. The development of this type of provider agency in turn can generate political support for the program.

A potential pitfall in the system is failure to plan and build in mechanisms that hold providers regularly accountable for the service delivered, in order to earn the advance payments. But careful design of the fiscal system required under the terms of the contract, together with technical assistance in developing vendor fiscal management capacity and a plan for gradual removal of the advance payment system, can overcome such problems. Then the system can be seen as serving its real purpose—encouraging the entry of small community-based organizations into the provider market and helping them reach the stage of development where they no longer require this extra level of financial support.

11

Addressing Management Issues

Part I of this book outlined a number of issues and themes in home care management. The case studies presented in the preceding five chapters of Part II address many of these concerns, drawing on the experience of some of the more advanced and innovative programs in the field. These programs, of course, are only five of many programs around the country that have developed their own solutions to home care management problems. Practices in other jurisdictions, though not studied in nearly as much detail by this project, shed further light on the themes and models described herein. These practices can be discussed in relation to six of the major management tasks of agencies funding home care: (1) allocation and targeting of resources, (2) program integration, (3) cost determination and rate setting, (4) maintaining adequate cash flow to providers, (5) monitoring fiscal and service performance, and (6) implementing appropriate management information and fiscal control systems.

ALLOCATION AND TARGETING OF RESOURCES

In allocating home care dollars and labor resources among different parts of a state and to individual clients, it is vitally important to match available dollars with the need for service. Finding an objective and valid means of making such a distribution can be difficult.

Maryland's Social Services Administration has tackled the problem of allocating its home care dollars and state-employed home aides among its counties by means of a "zero-based budget." With the help of a task force including representatives of local departments and vendors, a formula for distributing resources has been developed. The different factors that may indicate the potential need for services in the counties are weighted according to their importance. The formula is then used to calculate a total weighted need, at six-month intervals, for each county in the state. Resources are allocated accordingly. The formula, which is reviewed annually and is published, has apparently been found valid and reliable by the counties. New York State's Department of Social Services has also developed a formula for allocating Medicaid home care hours across the state.

At the local level, as the Alameda County example shows (Chapter 6), attention is increasingly focused on targeting dollars to those most in need of service and trying to insure that clients with comparable levels of need are allocated a similar level of resources. Programs operating within fixed budgets, as Alameda County's does, have particularly high stakes in the efficient and equitable allocation of resources to clients.

A number of other home care programs have also developed assessment tools that focus on the client's functional capacities in activities of everyday life (as opposed to medical data) and on the social supports available. These assessment data convert to an overall score. Washington, Texas, Illinois, Oregon, and Maryland all have reported the use of this type of assessment. In Washington and Illinois the score determines the maximum level of service the client may be allocated. In Illinois's Title XIX Community Care program, the service level is defined in terms of the maximum allowable monthly cost. In Washington it is defined in terms of the maximum number of hours per month. The average number of chore service hours per client dropped significantly in Washington after the standard assessment practice was introduced. In Texas the score determines what programs a client is eligible for and guides determination of the service hours a client will receive under the respective programs. Maryland's score is a measure of the risk of institutionalization and is used in different ways by different counties.

Case management as practiced in Connecticut's Promotion of Independent Living program and the Basic Channeling[1] demonstrations also is a method of targeting service resources. On the basis of a functional assessment, the case manager matches client need with the appropriate community service. The case manager identifies other resources that may be used to help pay for or provide the needed services, thereby using the Department on Aging's limited funds to leverage other funding sources.

PROGRAM INTEGRATION

One of the problems confronting home care programs is fragmentation of services. Much of this stems from the multiplicity of funding streams and public agencies responsible for in-home services, each with its own set of program constraints and administrative requirements. Because of fragmentation, clients requiring services may have to go to more than one agency before finding the agency operating the program for which they qualify and providing the services they need. Or, the services clients receive can be limited to those for which they are income eligible, which may not meet all their service needs. Similarly, providers serving clients under more than one program may have separate contracts and separate claims systems for each program under which they deliver services. Several methods are being used by different states and localities to address this problem area. To a degree the methods reflect the organizational structures and settings of the agencies, but the methods used generally fall into two models for the integration of home care programs. One model focuses on coordinating various service programs on behalf of the client; the other addresses the consolidation of administrative function for two or more home care programs.

[1]Basic Channeling demonstration programs funded by the Department of Health and Human Services to test approaches to minimizing the need for institutional care by channeling clients to appropriate community-based and other services.

The former approach is what Connecticut employs in its Promotion of Independent Living program and in the Basic Channeling demonstrations. This approach, which is also the basis of Case Coordination Units in Illinois, seeks to integrate home care services through a comprehensive model of case management in which the case manager coordinates a range of services required from different programs and agencies. No change is required in the fiscal and client management functions of programs operating under different funding streams. Instead, the case manager navigates and coordinates the funding streams as necessary to make up the service package appropriate to each client.

Several agencies indicate they are emphasizing integration of administrative tasks and responsibilities. The various functions that are integrated, however, vary widely. Texas uses a single set of case managers for eligibility, assessment, and client management for both its Title XX and Medicaid home care programs. Based on eligibility and assessment, the case manager decides under which program a client will receive services and, based on that determination, follows the appropriate procedure for identifying a provider. In Washington, the Area Agencies on Aging (AAA's) have the contractual responsibility for in-home services financed under Title III of the Older Americans Act (OAA) as well as for the Chore Services program, which is funded from state revenues and the Social Services Block Grant. Some of the AAA's in Oregon administer not only OAA and state revenues, but also Social Services Block Grant (SSBG) and Medicaid funds for long-term care. In cases where the AAA's have opted not to administer all long-term care dollars, the state's Senior Services Division administers SSBG and Medicaid funds.

Pennsylvania's Department of the Aging administers OAA, state, and SSBG dollars for the elderly. In 1982, the department folded all these funds into a single Aging Services Block Grant, which is allocated to the state's 50 AAA's. This eliminates the need for the AAA's to report and account separately for each funding stream. Instead, they maintain a single set of accounts on which they report. The state distributes expenditures to the various funding sources on the basis of uniform cost centers. Categorical program requirements are met through setting spending parameters for cost centers. Because the categorical requirements are met statewide, rather than at the local level, AAA's have greater program flexibility. At the same time, the system also increases fiscal control at the state level.

South Dakota's Department of Social Services administers home care programs funded through Medicaid, Title III, and the SSBG, while the state's Department of Health administers Medicare home health services. The two departments are the direct-service providers statewide. To avoid duplication of effort, they have a contractual arrangement whereby the Department of Health's community health nurses provide whatever nursing services are needed by the Department of Social Services and the Department of Social Services provides any aides needed by the Medicare program. The two agencies put their respective clients' data into a single computerized fiscal management system. Data from aides' time sheets is also put into the computer and checked against the client data. The computer then distributes the time spent to the various funding sources. This is used for both reporting and reimbursement.

Vermont has integrated some of its home care programs by pooling its funding sources and putting them through the Department of Health, and by consolidating the budgeting, planning, and administrative functions for the three main programs in the department. The department negotiates with the Home Health Assembly—a consortium of the home health agencies in the state which provide homemaker and home health services—to set formulas for allocation of the total SSBG and Vermont Annual Fund home health dollars among the agencies. The department then writes contracts with the individual agencies for case management and delivery of its programs. In this system, the home health agency is the single point of contact of the client. When service has been delivered, the home health agencies bill the Department of Health, which either draws resources from its line-item allocation for the SSBG or General Fund, or seeks Medicaid or Medicare reimbursement from the appropriate agency. As a check on home health agencies, the Department of Health reviews all assessments and audits all bills.

COST DETERMINATION AND RATE SETTING

Basic to sound fiscal management of any service is knowing what it costs to provide it. However, determining what home care services actually cost can be complicated if all the parties involved are not working with the same definition of cost. Chapter 3 took a detailed look at unit costs, one of the key issues involved in cost analysis, and at the uses to which managers can put cost information. Here we will summarize reports from a number of states on their efforts to deal with other aspects of the cost determination problem.

When it began contracting out the Chore Services program, Washington State established a statewide definition of its chore services as well as a standard unit of cost and standard cost reports to be used by AAA's in chore service contracts. This has enabled the state agency to get comparable information from localities across the state on chore service costs.

Pennsylvania's Department on Aging has also addressed the issue of what homemaker, chore, and home health service costs are in its program. In order to assure that it was getting uniform information on service costs from its AAA's, it issued an accounting manual in 1982 which defined cost centers and units of service and explained how indirect costs are to be treated. Pennsylvania reports that, since the accounting manual was issued, the cost data it receives have steadily improved. This has facilitated analysis of costs based on reports received through the state's management information system.

Contracting for the provision of home care services is a significant activity in many programs. Where this is the case, cost determination is a necessary part of rate setting. Three states that report using prospective or fixed unit rates (Washington, Texas, and Georgia) all negotiate rates on the basis of standardized cost reports from providers. New York City has used a two-tiered line-item cost reimbursement system.

The Arkansas Department of Human Sevices reports that it recently conducted a market survey and used this as the basis for setting the maximum allowable rate it will pay for home health services under Medicaid. Arkansas sought cost data independent of provider cost reports because it was changing its method of establishing the maximum rate. It had been using the Medicare maximum for its Medicaid program but decided that, because Medicare rates were based on reimbursing providers for *all* costs, they were inflationary. Hence, Arkansas used a market survey to determine what the direct costs were in the state and then factored in an additional percentage for indirect costs. Rates set using this approach were significantly lower than Medicare rates.

Because salaries and benefit levels are the main component of home care costs, the issue of pay levels and staff overhead is significant in cost comparison, not simply among individual providers but also across different provider systems, such as public employees, nonprofit agencies, and proprietary agencies. New Jersey reports that under its AFDC Homemaker/Home Health Aide demonstration, participating agencies have been allowed to set wages and hours according to the prevailing practices in their local communities. The state tracks those cost differentials to see how they relate to the retention rate of aides. The retention rate increased with increasing salary. As noted in Chapter 4, wage rates for aides need to be high enough in relation to employment markets so that excessive turnover is avoided.

MAINTAINING ADEQUATE CASH FLOW

For home care administrators whose programs provide services through contractual arrangements with service providers in the community, a fiscal problem that can arise is that of cash flow. When New York City's Office of Home Care decided to contract its program out to community-based organizations (some of which were newly created for this purpose), it designed a reimbursement system specifically to deal with the cash flow issue during the first years of vendorization. It developed a two-tiered reimbursement structure separating direct and indirect costs. To assure that agencies had the cash to pay aides' salaries, an advance payment was made for direct costs based upon a percentage of authorized service hours.

AAA's in the State of Washington have also on occasion confronted the same problem. There, however, state law prohibits the government from making advance payments to other than public bodies, so it has been necessary to evolve innovative ways of dealing with the problem, such as are described in Chapter 9. Maine makes provision for monthly advances based on budgeted expenses. As in New York, there is a year-end settlement against actual expenditures.

MONITORING FISCAL AND SERVICE PERFORMANCE

Sound fiscal management is increasingly seen to extend beyond the control of expenditures, to efficiency and quality of the program. In home care as in other fields, there is an increasing level of concern with fiscal and service performance. Previous chapters have already discussed the introduction of performance-based contracting in Texas, Washington, and Connecticut. New York City's Department for the Aging has also moved to performance contracts for its Title III program. Its contractors determined the actual service costs that would serve as the basis for negotiating a performance budget for the subsequent year.

In all of these cases the addition of performance standards to contracts has been used to assure a measure of control over services. Where contracts are on a fixed-price unit-rate basis, performance standards have provided the administering agency with a method for enforcing compliance with service expectations, substituting performance control for line-item or actual cost control. Monitoring performance against goals is a key part of program and financial reporting.

Failure to comply with standards on the part of a contractor can result in withholding of contract payments in Connecticut, termination of contracts in Washington, or prohibition to compete for the subsequent contract period in Texas. Incorporating reporting requirements and procedures in the contract to enable the contracting agency to monitor the contractor against the goals is central to these processes.

Pennsylvania's Department for the Aging has improved its capacity to monitor its AAA's fiscal and service performance by computer analysis of cost data from its management information system. The analysis enables the state to review the range of unit costs for a given service across the state and to identify the AAA's that are on the high or low side of the normal cost and service utilization range. Accountants are sent to those agencies to identify the cause of the variance. The AAA can then be offered additional technical assistance as necessary. The Iowa Department of Health has also used information from a statewide cost analysis as the basis for technical assistance efforts.

New Jersey uses independent professional reviews (IPR's) in its AFDC Homemaker/Home Health Aide project. The IPR team reviews the eligibility of the client and makes home visits to 20 percent of the clients in the project. The IPR's have found 5 or 6% of those evaluated ineligible under the policies governing the project. The home visits check on the quality of service being provided.

IMPLEMENTING MANAGEMENT AND FISCAL CONTROL SYSTEMS

Improving management's capacity to control program expenditures and to monitor the fiscal status of home care programs is at the heart of the efforts of many agencies to improve their information system and data bases. The introduction of computers to link various data bases and to perform fiscal functions is a recent feature in many of these programs. Alameda County's budget forecasting, described in Chapter 6, is an example.

One of the major areas in which home care programs have sought to improve their controls is in accounting. As concern about fraud and abuse has increased and as the size of programs has grown, some agencies have sought to improve control of program expenditures by developing systems to assure that payments are made only within authorized limits. Bills for services under the Arkansas Personal Care Program are handled through a computerized payment system that contains information on the units of service authorized for clients. The computer edits the bills, so payment is only generated for authorized units of service. New York City's Home Attendant Program uses a similar editing process.

Illinois, Michigan, and Missouri also report payment systems that edit claims or bills for authorized services; however, their systems (like those in Texas and Connecticut) have more edits than that in Arkansas. Illinois's payment system contains controls for client eligibility, client-specific vendor and service limits, and deductions of fees for which clients are responsible. Michigan's payment system controls for client authorizations, provider certification and rates, and client cost sharing. Missouri's prior authorization system edits bills for service, provider, time period, and units authorized.

Improvement of management information has been a major subject of innovations across the country. In some instances, the improved information approaches have evolved from existing management information systems; in others, from accounting systems. Computer technology has been used to link formerly separate data bases, thereby expanding the capacity to use information for a variety of purposes.

By coding the state chart of accounts, Maryland's Social Service Administration has improved its record keeping on program expenditures without adding to the reporting requirements of its counties. Accounting codes categorize expenditures by county, type of expenditure, and type of provider. The monthly expenditure report produced by the state fiscal office, based on the chart of accounts, enables program managers to track purchase of service dollars. By cross-referencing the expenditure report with monthly client information reports from counties, the cost per unit of service can be tracked.

Pennsylvania's Department on Aging puts financial reports and data from its AAA programs into its management information system. It can then analyze average unit costs by service, average units of service, and average cost per person across the state. This information is used both for planning purposes and for comparing the cost efficiency of the various AAA's across the state.

The Missouri Department of Social Services and the Illinois Department on Aging have developed the capacity to link their computerized client data base and their Medicaid management information system. This enables them to track all Medicaid costs and services utilization for long-term care clients. Missouri plans to add Social Service Block Grant client and expenditure data so that social service costs and utilization, as well as Medicaid service utilization, can be tracked.

A variation on the system where budget control measures are linked to an accounting system is one where budget control is linked to client care planning. In federally funded "Complex Channeling" demonstrations where there were caps on client service costs, there was a special need for the projects to control service dollar authorizations and payments. To meet this need a client-related financial control system was developed by an accounting firm (Arthur Young and Company) working on the nationwide demonstration effort. The system, which is partially automated, fulfills the functions of budget preparation, client care plan cost calculation, client payment requirements, service order authorization, provider reimbursement, and fiscal status reporting. The system is not an accounting system, but data from the client fiscal control system are used as input to the accounting system. Complex Channeling sites have included Miami, Florida; Lynn, Massachusetts; Troy, New York; Cleveland, Ohio; and Philadelphia, Pennsylvania.

The OnLok Senior Health Services program in San Francisco, another demonstration project in comprehensive community care, has developed a management information system that integrates both its fiscal and client information systems through a multiuser microcomputer. The integrated system was developed from a provider perspective and meets the programs' operational, policy, and research needs. The fiscal component of the system is a comprehensive cash management system that incorporates payroll, billing, accounts payable, fixed assets depreciation, and the general ledger. The payroll program can distribute individual salaries to different funding sources through the general ledger, which allows reporting by type of expense, cost center, and funding source. The client management component incorporates the client master system, service data, and assessment data. The client system provides clinical information (i.e., service scheduling, staff load monitoring, progress recording) on a day-to-day basis and produces routine management reports. The system automatically integrates cost and service information, enabling periodical tracking of unit costs and ongoing tracking of total service costs by program participant.

One of the problems for agencies employing home health aides is processing the workers' time sheets for billing and reimbursement purposes, often for multiple funding sources. Two agencies reported that they have developed systems for processing time sheets more efficiently. Aides working for South Dakota's Department of Social Services complete time studies accounting for 100 percent of their time, identifying clients served, type of service provided, travel time, mileage, and administrative time. The information from the time studies is entered into a computer and used for reimbursement purposes.

Most of the approaches described in this section rely on computers. Another technological advance that has not yet been applied to home care but may come along in the future is the use of bar code identification cards to track client service utilization. These can be used in combination with a bar code reader and Apple® computer to generate sources. The Aging Services Division in Phoenix, Arizona is now using this technology at its nutrition sites.

CONCLUSION AND FUTURE DIRECTIONS

The development of a more comprehensive set of home care systems, with substantial federal support, can appropriately be seen as a major "sleeper issue" in American social policy. A variety of indicators suggest that need and demand for such a system will be on the increase in coming years. Only 5 to 6 percent of Americans over age 65 are utilizing nursing homes or other long-term institutional care at any given time; yet the cost of their care was $30 billion per year in 1984 and can be estimated at more than $35 billion per year for 1987 (Waldo, Levit, & Lazenby, 1986). Although it appears that the typical level of impairment among nursing home residents is increasing (Hing, 1987), it is still the case that many persons, particularly in areas of the country without extensive home care programs, receive nursing home care who could be cared for more satisfactorily at home. It has been shown by the experience of programs like the New York home care program that even very severely impaired patients, including the incontinent, the nonambulatory, and those who are almost totally dependent in personal care, can be cared for at home. Even specialized therapies such as total parenteral nutrition are increasingly being administered at home. The nonelderly disabled, including persons with extreme dependence in activities of daily living, are more and more often demanding their right to liberation from chronic-care hospitals and other long-term-care facilities, in order to live in a home environment. They are joining with advocates for the elderly as a strong constituency demanding more widespread availability of home care.

European experience, too, indicates that in-home care can be the principal care modality for a much higher proportion of long-term-care clients than is yet the case in the United States. In Great Britain, for example, institutional bed supplies are limited: An estimated 3.9 percent of elderly received institutional care in 1980, less than three-quarters of the U.S. rate for that year. Concurrently, public home care is relied on much more heavily than in the United States; the proportion of elderly receiving home care is more than twice the U.S. rate (U.S. Senate, 1984).

Cost control efforts in other sectors of the long-term-care system also add to pressures on home care. Up until the 1980s, hospitals served a significant, if usually unheralded, function as long-term-care providers of last resort, with many hospitals caring for hard-to-place patients for much longer than the need for acute care persisted. Such patients accounted for as many as one-quarter of the beds, or even more at some urban hospitals. The advent of the DRG system created, really for the first time, an operational as well as theoretical definition of the role of hospitals in the United States as places for acute, curative care only, and it significantly increased pressures on home care programs. Concurrently, the success of state policy initiatives to restrict use of nursing homes under Medicaid to those with the greatest care needs pushed many individuals with only moderate impairments out of that system. This was perhaps appropriate, but these patients still needed care of some kind. Public policies at the state level generally constrained increases in nursing home supply during the late 1970s and 1980s to a rate below the growth in the at-risk population.

Finally, while the numbers of the very old in the population increased, other social trends reduced the availability of the family and other informal supports that had traditionally been the care source for the majority of functionally impaired elderly and disabled. Improvements in the economic status of the elderly made it possible for more and more of them to act on what appears to have been their long-standing preference for establishing their own, separate households. One result has been that, when impairment increased, care from within the household was less likely to be available. As married women in their middle years have increasingly participated in the labor force, they have become less likely to be available as caretakers for elderly relatives. Depending on the definition used, somewhere around 10 percent of the noninstitutionalized elderly have functional impairments that limit their ability to perform basic activities of daily living without help; this number is larger than the total number of institutionalized elderly. The predominant source of care for these individuals currently is family assistance, not formal home care; but, as the social trends just discussed continue, there will be increased need that cannot be met through informal sources and is unlikely to be met through institutional expansion and probably should not be met through that route.

It has been fairly widely noted that a concatenation of social forces is increasing demand for formal long-term care. It also needs to be noted that expansion of institutional care in order to meet this demand fully does not appear to be in the cards; in fact, the growth rate in bed supply that was apparent in the late 1960s and early 1970s has subsequently been constrained, largely by deliberate public policies such as Certificate of Need limits and reimbursement restrictions. Further, there is strong evidence that almost any viable alternative is preferred to a nursing home by the potential consumers of such care themselves. For all these reasons, strong demand for growth in home care programs can be expected to continue, both at the political level and in terms of increasing numbers of claimants for service.

In the current tax-limitation environment, which can be expected to continue for some years, programs such as home care that are experiencing growth in demand can expect to come under extreme pressure to show (1) that they are capable of efficient, cost-effective management, particularly with respect to fiscal functions; (2) that they can allocate resources in a way that is defensible and equitable; and (3) that they have the wherewithal to document who it is they are serving and at what cost. Service allocation decisions, for example, will undergo increasing scrutiny, and systems like the Alameda County model will be the subject of careful attention, as indicated already by the statewide adoption of that system. As the sophisticated use of computer-based management information systems comes to be taken increasingly for granted elsewhere in government and in the private sector, agencies administering home care programs can count on being expected to use fiscal and programmatic data in an integrated fashion to monitor program performance. Computerization of previously manual functions offers an important, if often bypassed, opportunity to rethink information management requirements at a fundamental level, cross-link previously separate data, and use these cross-linked data to provide new dimensions of information and control. The purchase of services from direct-provider agencies, too, is increasingly becoming accepted across a variety of government functions, and ad hoc or casual approaches to establishing and managing such contractual relationships are becoming less acceptable.

It is not too much to hope that, in providing long-term care, we will begin to think of nursing homes as an alternative to home care, rather than the other way around. Implementing home care more widely—at a satisfactory level of adequacy and as a basic entitlement for the disabled and the impaired elderly—is a badly needed reform in American social policy. The successful growth of these programs, however, requires careful attention to the management issues described in this book; thus, these are not simply narrow technical issues but critical problems that must be addressed as policy reforms are undertaken.

References

American Public Welfare Association. (1982). *Public Welfare Directory, 1982/1983*. Washington, DC: American Public Welfare Association.

Bishop, C., & Stassen, M. (1986). Prospective reimbursement for home health care. *Pride Institute Journal of Home Health Care, 5* (1), 18–19.

Burwell, B. (1986). *Shared obligations: Public policy influences on family care for the elderly* (Medicaid Program Evaluation Working Paper 2.1). Washington, DC: Health Care Financing Administration.

Crystal, S. (1984). *America's old age crisis: Public policy and the two worlds of aging* (Rev. ed.). New York: Basic Books.

Doty, P., Liu, K., & Wiener, J. (1985). An overview of long-term care. *Health Care Financing Review, 6* (3), 69–78.

Frost & Sullivan. (1983). *Home healthcare products and services: Markets in the U.S.* New York: Frost and Sullivan.

Ginzberg, E., Balinsky, W., & Ostow, M. (1984). *Home health care, its role in the changing health services market.* Totowa, NJ: Rowman and Allanheld.

Hayes, F., Grossman, D., Thomas, J., & Mechling, J. (1982). *Linkages: Improving financial management in local government.* Washington, DC: Urban Institute Press.

Hing, E. (1987, May). Use of nursing homes by the elderly: Preliminary data from the 1985 National Nursing Home Survey. *Advance Data for Vital and Health Statistics,* No. 135. Hyattsville, MD: National Center for Health Statistics.

Hughes, S. (1986). *Long-term care: Options in an expanding market.* Homewood, IL: Dow Jones—Irwin.

Kane, R. (1985). Long-term care status quo untenable? What is more ideal for nation's elderly? *Perspective on Aging, 14* (5), 23–26.

Layzer, E. (1981). *Individual providers in home care: Their practice, problems, and implications in the delivery of homemaker-home health aide services.* New York: National HomeCaring Council.

Leader, S. (1986, September). Home health benefits under Medicare (AARP Public Policy Institute Report Number 8601). Washington, DC: American Association of Retired Persons.

Nassif, J. (1985). *The home health care solution.* New York: Harper and Row.

National HomeCaring Council. (1980). *Model curriculum for home-maker–home health aides.* New York: Author.

National Research Council. (1985). *Women's work, men's work: Sex segregation on the job.* Washington, DC: National Academy Press.

Oriol, W. (1985). *The complex cube of long-term care.* Washington, DC: American Health Planning Association.

Reif, L., & Trager, B. (Eds). (1985). *International perspectives on long-term care.* New York: Haworth Press.

Schick, A. (1966, December). The road to PPB. *Public Administration Review.*

Shinn, E. (1984). *Handbook for computing the cost of an hour of direct homemaker—home health aide service.* New York: National HomeCaring Council.

Silverberg, G. (1984). *Employment determinations and unemployment compensation in supportive home care.* Madison, WI: Department of Health and Social Services.

Terlizzi, L. (1977). *Human resources issues in the field of aging: Home-maker—home health aide services* (AOA Occasional Papers in Gerontology, No. 2). Washington, DC: Department of Health, Education and Welfare (DHEW Publication No. OHD 77–20086).

United States Senate. (1984, July). *Long-term care in Western Europe and Canada: Implications for the United States* (Special Committee on Aging, Information Paper, Senate Print 98–211). Washington, DC: U.S. Government Printing Office.

Urban Systems Research and Engineering. (1982). *In-home services and the contribution of kin: Substitution effects in home care programs for the elderly* (Final report, Contract No. HHS-100-81-0-026). Cambridge, MA: Urban Systems Research and Engineering.

Waldo, D., Levit, K., & Lazenby, H. (1986). National health expenditures, 1985. *Health Care Financing Review, 8*(1), 1–21.

Weisman, J. (1985, August). New York State home attendant regulations: Mostly bad news. *Monthly Report* (pp. 4–5). New York: Eastern Paralyzed Veterans' Association.

Weissert, W. (1985a). Seven reasons why it is so difficult to make community-based long-term care cost effective. *Journal of Health Services Research, 20*(3).

Weissert, W. (1985b). Estimating the long-term care population: Prevalence rates and selected characteristics. *Health Care Financing Review, 6*(4), 83–91.

Wood, B., & Rosen, C. (1980). *Title XX in California: A study of social services for adults* (Staff Study, USDHHS Regional Office). San Francisco: U.S. Department of Health and Human Services.

Index

Index

Springer Publishing Company

Long-Term Care
Principles, Programs, and Policies
Rosalie A. Kane and **Robert Kane**
Presents a thorough overview of current long-term care systems. Integrating extensive data about nursing home care, day care, foster care, respite care, and case management, the authors analyse the organization, functioning, and effects of these systems on their specific target populations. Valuable for students and administrators. 432pp / 1987

Stroke in the Elderly
New Issues in Diagnosis, Treatment, and Rehabilitation
Ruth Dunkle and **James Schmidley,** *Editors*
This multidisciplinary volume provides information on the most recent scientific approaches to the care of the older stroke victim within three major categories: risk factors, treatment, and rehabilitation. Any practitioner involved with aging and health care will find this book of interest. 224pp / 1987

Managing Home Care for the Elderly
Anabel O. Pelham and **William F. Clark,** *Editors*
These studies document important recent experiments in providing care at home for the elderly. Contributors discuss case management approaches, the provision of supplementary services and other key topics. 208pp / 1985

Communication Skills for Working with Elders
Barbara B. Dreher
This book provides a practical guide to effective interaction with the elderly and presents techniques for overcoming common communication problems and disorders found among aging persons. Emphasizing skills development, the author explores the physical, social, and emotional changes that can create unique communication needs. 160pp / 1987

A Basic Guide to Working With Elders
Michael J. Salamon
Describes specific techniques for such common tasks as interviewing older adults, assessing needs, and designing programs. Comprehensive and extremely practical, the book is also appropriate for the instruction of students involved in gerontology and geriatrics. 224pp / 1986

Exercise Activities for the Elderly
Kay Flatten, Barbara Wilhite, and **Eleanor Reyes-Watson**
Here is a handy resource for those working directly with institutionalized and home-bound elders. A variety of exercises is presented, some of which are geared to clients with such conditions as arthritis and diabetes, and others which are designed to build up muscular strength and maintain flexibility. 224pp / 1987

Recreation Activities for the Elderly
Kay Flatten, Barbara Wilhite, and **Eleanor Reyes-Watson**
Included in this guide are simple crafts that utilize easily obtainable, inexpensive materials and hobbies focusing on collections, nature, and the arts for home-bound and institutionalized elders. 240pp / 1987

Order from your bookdealer or directly from publisher.

Springer Publishing Co. 536 Broadway, New York, New York 10012

B15